Alcohol and Substance Abuse in Older Adults

Editors

RITA KHOURY
GEORGE T. GROSSBERG

CLINICS IN GERIATRIC MEDICINE

www.geriatric.theclinics.com

February 2022 • Volume 38 • Number 1

ELSEVIER

1600 John F. Kennedy Boulevard • Suite 1800 • Philadelphia, Pennsylvania, 19103-2899

http://www.theclinics.com

CLINICS IN GERIATRIC MEDICINE Volume 38, Number 1
February 2022 ISSN 0749–0690, ISBN-13: 978-0-323-84999-9

Editor: Katerina Heidhausen
Developmental Editor: Hannah Almira Lopez

Clinics in Geriatric Medicine (ISSN 0749-0690) is published quarterly by Elsevier Inc., 360 Park Avenue South, New York, NY 10010-1710. Months of issue are February, May, August, and November. Business and Editorial Offices: 1600 John F. Kennedy Blvd., Suite 1800, Philadelphia, PA 191023-2899. Periodicals postage paid at New York, NY, and additional mailing offices. Subscription prices are $303.00 per year (US individuals), $901.00 per year (US institutions), $100.00 per year (US & Canadian student/resident), $330.00 per year (Canadian individuals), $928.00 per year (Canadian institutions), $431.00 per year (international individuals), $928.00 per year (international institutions), and $195.00 per year (international student/resident). Foreign air speed delivery is included in all *Clinics* subscription prices. All prices are subject to change without notice. POSTMASTER: Send address changes to *Clinics in Geriatric Medicine,* Elsevier Health Sciences Division, Subscription Customer Service, 3251 Riverport Lane, Maryland Heights, MO 63043. **Telephone: 1-800-654-2452 (U.S. and Canada); 314-447-8871 (outside U.S. and Canada). Fax: 314-447-8029. E-mail:** journalscustomerservice-usa@elsevier.com **(for print support)** or journalsonlinesupport-usa@elsevier.com **(for online support).**

Reprints. For copies of 100 or more, of articles in this publication, please contact the Commercial Reprints Department, Elsevier Inc., 360 Park Avenue South, New York, New York 10010-1710. Tel.: 212-633-3874; Fax: 212-633-3820, E-mail: reprints@elsevier.com.

Clinics in Geriatric Medicine is covered in *MEDLINE/PubMed (Index Medicus), EMBASE/Excerpta Medica, Current Contents/Clinical Medicine (CC/CM),* and the *Cumulative Index to Nursing & Allied Health Literature.*

Contributors

EDITORS

RITA KHOURY, MD
Assistant Professor, Geriatric Psychiatrist, Department of Psychiatry and Clinical Psychology, Saint Georges Hospital University Medical Center, University of Balamand, Faculty of Medicine, Beirut, Lebanon; Adjunct Faculty, Department of Psychiatry and Behavioral Neuroscience, Saint Louis University School of Medicine, St Louis, Missouri, USA

GEORGE T. GROSSBERG, MD
Professor, Geriatric Psychiatrist, Department of Psychiatry and Behavioral Neuroscience, Division of Geriatric Psychiatry, Saint Louis University School of Medicine, St Louis, Missouri, USA

AUTHORS

VICTORIA AHMAD, MD
University of Balamand, Faculty of Medicine, Saint Georges Hospital University Medical Center, Beirut, Lebanon

ESRA ATES BULUT, MD
Associate Professor, Department of Geriatric Medicine, Adana City Training and Research Hospital, Adana, Turkey

NAZEM K. BASSIL, MD
Associate Professor of Clinical Medicine, Geriatric Medicine, Palliative Care, Balamand University, Saint George Hospital University Medical Center, Beirut, Lebanon

THEODORA G. BOU SABA, MD
Resident, Family Medicine, Balamand University, Saint George Hospital University Medical Center, Beirut, Lebanon

NICOLE BRANDT, PharmD, MBA, BCGP, BCPP, FASCP
Executive Director, The Peter Lamy Center on Drug Therapy and Aging; Professor, University of Maryland School of Pharmacy; Clinical Pharmacist, MedStar Center for Successful Aging

DEREK BROWN, MD
Department of Psychiatry and Behavioral Neuroscience, Division of Geriatric Psychiatry, Saint Louis University School of Medicine, St Louis, Missouri, USA

ELISABETH C. DEMARCO, BS
Department of Psychiatry and Behavioral Neuroscience, Division of Geriatric Psychiatry, Saint Louis University School of Medicine, St Louis, Missouri, USA

ABHILASH DESAI, MD
Adjunct Associate Professor, Division of Geriatric Psychiatry, Department of Psychiatry, Saint Louis University School of Medicine; Adjunct Associate Professor, Department of Psychiatry and Behavioral Sciences, University of Washington School of Medicine

RAJAT DUGGIRALA, MD
Psychiatry Resident, Saint Louis University, St Louis, Missouri, USA

HUSSEIN EL BOURJI, BS
Faculty of Medicine, American University of Beirut, Beirut, Lebanon

TAMARA KADI, BA
Faculty of Medicine, American University of Beirut, Beirut, Lebanon

SAMER EL HAYEK, MD
Department of Psychiatry, American University of Beirut, Beirut, Lebanon

LUNA GEAGEA, MD
Department of Psychiatry, American University of Beirut, Beirut, Lebanon

ZIAD GHANTOUS, MD
University of Balamand, Faculty of Medicine, Saint Georges Hospital University Medical Center, Beirut, Lebanon

ELIAS GHOSSOUB, MD, MSc
Department of Psychiatry, American University of Beirut, Beirut, Lebanon

GEORGE T. GROSSBERG, MD
Professor, Geriatric Psychiatrist, Department of Psychiatry and Behavioral Neuroscience, Division of Geriatric Psychiatry, Saint Louis University School of Medicine, St Louis, Missouri, USA

HEIDI HOFFMAN, MD
Saint Louis University School of Medicine, Saint Louis University, St Louis, Missouri, USA

ROY IBRAHIM, BS
Third Year Medical Student, Faculty of Medicine, University of Balamand, Beirut, Lebanon

AHMET TURAN ISIK, MD
Professor, Unit for Aging Brain and Dementia, Department of Geriatric Medicine, Faculty of Medicine, Dokuz Eylul University, Izmir, Turkey

CHANCHAL KAHLON, BS
Saint Louis University School of Medicine, Saint Louis University, St Louis, Missouri, USA

RITA KHOURY, MD
Assistant Professor of Clinical Psychiatry, Geriatric Psychiatrist, Department of Psychiatry and Clinical Psychology, Saint Georges Hospital University Medical Center, University of Balamand, Faculty of Medicine, Beirut, Lebanon; Adjunct Faculty, Department of Psychiatry and Behavioral Neuroscience, Saint Louis University School of Medicine, St Louis Missouri, USA

SUNIL KHUSHALANI, MD, DFAPA, FASAM
Chief Medical Officer, Kolmac Outpatient Recovery Centers, Burtonsville, Maryland, USA

ELLEN KIM, MD
Department of Psychiatry and Behavioral Neuroscience, Resident Physician in Psychiatry, Saint Louis University School of Medicine, St Louis, Missouri, USA

GABRIELA FENOLLAL-MALDONADO, MD
Department of Psychiatry and Behavioral Neuroscience, Division of Geriatric Psychiatry, Saint Louis University School of Medicine, St Louis, Missouri, USA

PETER MALIHA, MD
Second year Psychiatry Resident, Department of Psychiatry and Clinical Psychology, Saint Georges Hospital University Medical Center, Faculty of Medicine, University of Balamand, Beirut, Lebanon

BERNADETTE MDAWAR, MD
Department of Psychiatry, American University of Beirut, Beirut, Lebanon

BRIANNE M. NEWMAN, MD
Department of Psychiatry and Behavioral Neuroscience, Associate Professor, Saint Louis University School of Medicine, St Louis, Missouri, USA

MARIE LENA K. OHANIAN, MD
Resident, Family Medicine, Balamand University, Saint George Hospital University Medical Center, Beirut, Lebanon

TODD PALMER, MD
Director, Addiction Fellowship, Family Medicine Residency of Idaho, Boise, Idaho, USA

SAIF-UR-RAHMAN PARACHA, MD
Division of Geriatric Psychiatry, Department of Psychiatry and Behavioral Neuroscience, Saint Louis University School of Medicine, St Louis, Missouri, USA

WM MAURICE REDDEN, MD
Division of Geriatric Psychiatry, Department of Psychiatry and Behavioral Neuroscience, Saint Louis University School of Medicine, St Louis, Missouri, USA

NEIL M. ROBINSON
Medical Student, Saint Louis University School of Medicine, St Louis, Missouri, USA

MIRIAM B. RODIN, MD, PhD
Professor, Division of Geriatric Medicine, Geriatric Medicine Program Director, Department of Internal Medicine, Saint Louis University School of Medicine, SLUCare Academic Pavilion, St Louis, Missouri, USA

DELAVAR SAFARI, BA
Department of Psychiatry and Behavioral Neuroscience, Division of Geriatric Psychiatry, Saint Louis University School of Medicine, St Louis, Missouri, USA

LILLIAN SCANLON, BS
Department of Psychiatry and Behavioral Neuroscience, Division of Geriatric Psychiatry, Saint Louis University School of Medicine, St Louis, Missouri, USA

QURATULANNE SHEHERYAR, MD
Division of Geriatric Psychiatry, Department of Psychiatry and Behavioral Neuroscience, Saint Louis University School of Medicine, St Louis, Missouri, USA

FARID TALIH, MD
Department of Psychiatry, American University of Beirut, Beirut, Lebanon

Contents

Preface: Alcohol, Drugs, and Baby Boomers   xiii

Rita Khoury and George T. Grossberg

Alcohol Use Disorder in Older Adults   1

Gabriela Fenollal Maldonado, Derek Brown, Heidi Hoffman, Chanchal Kahlon, and George Grossberg

> As the number of older adults worldwide continues to increase, we observe a proportional growth of substance use. Despite the myriad of complications alcohol use disorder (AUD) has on the body, with regards to organ systems and mental health, the topic has been underresearched in the older adult population. Thus, it is important to create awareness about the growing problem of AUD among older adults. In this way, we can mitigate the long-term complications and side effects observed with alcohol abuse in this vulnerable population.

Screening for and Management of Opioid Use Disorder in Older Adults in Primary Care   23

Rajat Duggirala, Sunil Khushalani, Todd Palmer, Nicole Brandt, and Abhilash Desai

> Opioid use disorder (OUD) is commonly seen in older adults in primary care offices. OUD when left untreated, often leads to overdose deaths, emergency department visits, and hospitalizations due to opioid-related adverse effects, especially respiratory and central nervous system depression. Primary care providers are on the front lines of efforts for its prevention, early detection, and treatment. This includes using the lowest doses of opioids for the shortest possible time for management of pain, routine screening, brief intervention, opioid withdrawal management, prescription of naloxone to prevent overdose death, and treatment with medications and psychosocial interventions for OUD. Referral to addiction treatment centers may be needed in complex cases. This review explores the epidemiology, screening, as well as management of OUD as it pertains to the elderly population.

Illicit Drug Use in Older Adults: An Invisible Epidemic?   39

Ziad Ghantous, Victoria Ahmad, and Rita Khoury

> Illicit drug use/misuse among older adults is understudied, although current trends point to older adults being the fastest-growing segment in the United States and other developed countries. There is a need for further insight into drug use patterns in older adults, who face their own set of socioeconomic, medical, and psychiatric problems. We reviewed the literature for data related to use/misuse of heroin and stimulants (cocaine, amphetamines, and methamphetamines) among people over the age of 40 years. We focused on prevalence rates of use/misuse of these substances, comorbidities, diagnostic challenges, screening tools, and treatment recommendations specific to the geriatric population.

Hallucinogen Use and Misuse in Older Adults   55

Wm Maurice Redden, Saif-Ur-Rahman Paracha, and Quratulanne Sheheryar

Hallucinogens, or psychedelics, are substances/drugs that have been used for over a millennium. The most well known are LSD, psilocybin, mescaline, and PCP. These substances may induce hallucinations as well as cause somatic and psychological symptoms. Because of the Controlled Substances Act of 1970, there has been very little research done to determine the long-term consequences or perhaps potential benefit of misuse and abuse of hallucinogens. Typically, these drugs are not abused but more often misused. Recently, there has been a renewed interest in these compounds, which may lead to possible therapeutic options.

Cannabis Use and Misuse in Older Adults   67

Rita Khoury, Peter Maliha, and Roy Ibrahim

Cannabis is the most frequently used illegal psychoactive substance by older adults. With population aging, legalization and medicalization of cannabis, and changes in perceptions of older adults toward its use, recreational and medical cannabis use/misuse is on the rise in seniors. Although there are solid data related to the adverse events of cannabis in older adults, efficacy data are lacking. Older adults are at increased risk of developing cannabis use disorder alongside other medical and psychiatric comorbidities. We review the benefits and risks associated with cannabis use, and screening and management strategies for cannabis use disorder in older adults.

Abuse/Misuse of Prescription Medications in Older Adults   85

Esra Ates Bulut and Ahmet Turan ISIK

The world population is aging due to increasing life expectancy. The rate of drug use increases, and inappropriate prescribing is frequently encountered with advancing age. In addition, misuse and abuse of prescription drugs is a serious problem in older adults. It is challenging to detect substance and drug abuse in older patients because it may have fewer consequences in social, legal, and occupational fields. However, there is not enough information about the screening, evaluation, diagnosis, and treatment of abuse. Therefore, the awareness of health care professionals and others involved in older patients' care should be raised about the misuse and abuse of drugs.

Over-The-Counter Remedies in Older Adults: Patterns of Use, Potential Pitfalls, and Proposed Solutions   99

Delavar Safari, Elisabeth C. DeMarco, Lillian Scanlon, and George T. Grossberg

Over-the-counter (OTC) products such as pharmaceuticals, dietary supplements, vitamins, and herbal remedies are widely available and copiously used by older adults for health maintenance and symptom management. Owing to physiology, multimorbidity, and polypharmacy, this population is particularly vulnerable to inappropriate use of OTC products, adverse effects, and drug interactions. While OTC pharmaceuticals are bound by FDA-approved standards, dietary supplements are regulated differently, resulting in variable quality and increased possibility for adulteration. Internationally, standards for OTC products vary widely. Accessible educational information, improved provider–patient communication, and revision of regulatory policy could improve safety for older adult users of OTC products.

Nicotine Use Disorder in Older Adults   119
Nazem K. Bassil, Marie Lena K. Ohanian, and Theodora G. Bou Saba

Nicotine is one of the most abused substances worldwide. Just as in adolescence and adulthood, tobacco use is also problematic in the elderly. Older people are more vulnerable to smoking consequences because of the additive effects of smoke. Cardiovascular diseases are the most common health problems associated with smoking; however, other systems are also affected, including the respiratory, nervous, integumentary, and many other systems. Smoking cessation is a difficult task especially in the elderly; therefore, physicians should encourage older patients to quit with every patient-physician encounter by offering counseling and replacement therapy.

A Brewed Awakening: Neuropsychiatric Effects of Caffeine in Older Adults   133
Ellen Kim, Neil M. Robinson, and Brianne M. Newman

This article provides a current review of the literature examining caffeine use in older adults. Caffeine use is prevalent among older adults; thus, providers need to be aware of the prevalence and diagnostic criteria of caffeine use disorder versus nonproblematic use. The relationship between caffeine and various neuropsychiatric disorders, including Parkinson's disease, Alzheimer's disease, insomnia, and late-life depression, is reviewed. The neurobiological effects of caffeine are described, along with clinically relevant interactions between caffeine and common psychotropic medications.

Applying Geriatric Principles to Hazardous Drinking in Older Adults   145
Miriam B. Rodin

Older adults continue to drink as they age. Aging changes alcohol kinetics just as with any other drug. Older adults have increased sensitivity to acute alcohol intake that accounts for the increased risk of falls, traffic accidents, and other injury. The Annual Medicare Wellness Exam is an excellent opportunity to introduce screening for unsafe drinking along with accumulated risks and deficits of aging. Older adults have responded well to brief interventions for unhealthy drinking. In the presence of alcohol use disorder or serious comorbidity including psychiatric illness, referral to specialized multidisciplinary care can be lifesaving.

Substance Misuse and the Older Offender   159
Samer El Hayek, Bernadette Mdawar, and Elias Ghossoub

Substance misuse is prevalent among older adults involved in the criminal justice system. Older offenders are primarily defined as individuals 50 years and older. The different classes of older offenders and their offending behaviors vary in their association with substance misuse. Most prison healthcare systems do not adequately integrate substance use services. Screening for and treatment of substance misuse should be part of comprehensive mental health programs tailored to older offenders. This article reviews different types of offenses among older offenders, their association with substance misuse, as well as available treatment services.

Prevention Strategies of Alcohol and Substance Use Disorders in Older Adults   169

Samer El Hayek, Luna Geagea, Hussein El Bourji, Tamara Kadi, and Farid Talih

Older adults are increasingly engaging in unhealthy substance use. Owing to aging and comorbid medical conditions, older adults are at increased risk of adverse effects from alcohol, tobacco, and illicit drug use. Preventative measures, regular screening, and appropriate intervention can protect older adults from the negative outcomes of substance use and potentially improve their quality of life. This article reviews the latest trends of substance use in older adults, impact on health, and the best practice approaches for the clinical assessment of substance use disorders in this age group.

CLINICS IN GERIATRIC MEDICINE

FORTHCOMING ISSUES

May 2022
Osteoarthritis
David J. Hunter, *Editor*

August 2022
COVID-19 in the Geriatric Patient
Francesco Landi, *Editor*

RECENT ISSUES

November 2021
Women's Health
Karen A. Blackstone and Elizabeth L. Cobbs, *Editors*

August 2021
Sleep in the Elderly
Steven H. Feinsilver and Margarita Oks, *Editors*

SERIES OF RELATED INTEREST

Medical Clinics
https://www.medical.theclinics.com/
Primary Care: Clinics in Office Practice
https://www.primarycare.theclinics.com/

THE CLINICS ARE AVAILABLE ONLINE!
Access your subscription at:
www.theclinics.com

Preface

Alcohol, Drugs, and Baby Boomers

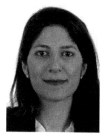 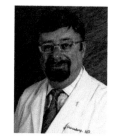

Rita Khoury, MD   George T. Grossberg, MD
Editors

There were 703 million persons aged 65 years or over in the world in 2019. The number of older persons is projected to double to 1.5 billion in 2050.[1]

Alcohol and substance use has been increasing in this population, notably with the aging of the "baby boomers," who were introduced to illicit substances in their late teens/early adulthood.

Due to their preexisting medical problems and physiologic changes experienced with age, older adults are at higher risk of developing medical and psychiatric adverse events due to their hazardous use of alcohol and different substances. Although there are no criteria specifically developed to define alcohol and substance use disorders in older adults, several screening and diagnostic tools have been developed or adapted for seniors. It is crucial to identify these disorders early and establish prompt treatment strategies to improve seniors' physical and mental health, as well as quality of life. Application of prevention strategies, notably by primary care physicians, is key to decreasing the societal burden of these disorders.

In this issue of *Clinics in Geriatric Medicine*, the epidemiology, screening, diagnosis, and treatments of alcohol and illicit substance use disorders in older adults are reviewed. Substances include cannabis, hallucinogens, cocaine, heroin and other opioids, stimulants, and other prescription medicines, over-the-counter medications, nicotine, and caffeine. Cooccurring medical and psychiatric comorbidities in older adults are also reviewed within each article. Management strategies are often multimodal, combining pharmacotherapy and psychosocial care.

Clin Geriatr Med 38 (2022) xiii–xiv
https://doi.org/10.1016/j.cger.2021.07.012
0749-0690/22/© 2021 Published by Elsevier Inc.

All articles have been written by international experts in the field and provide the latest scientific evidence to guide primary care physicians, geriatricians, and mental health care workers in the diagnosis and clinical decision making in older patients.

Rita Khoury, MD
Department of Psychiatry and
Clinical Psychology
Saint Georges Hospital University Medical Center
Youssef Sursock Street
PO Box 166378
Beirut, Lebanon

George T. Grossberg, MD
Department of Psychiatry and
Behavioral Neuroscience
Saint Louis University School of Medicine
Monteleone Hall
1438 South Grand Boulevard
St Louis, MO 63104, USA

E-mail addresses:
rita.khoury@idraac.org; rita.khoury.md@gmail.com (R. Khoury)
george.grossberg@health.slu.edu (G.T. Grossberg)

REFERENCE

1. United Nations. Department of Economic and Social Affairs, Population Division (2020). World Population Ageing 2019.

Alcohol Use Disorder in Older Adults

Gabriela Fenollal-Maldonado, MD[a],*, Derek Brown, MD[b], Heidi Hoffman, MD[c], Chanchal Kahlon, BS[d], George Grossberg, MD[e]

KEYWORDS

- Alcohol use • Geriatric • Elderly • Older adults

KEY POINTS

- Substance use in older adults is one of the fastest growing health problems in the United States
- Increased alcohol use adversely affects multiple aspects of one's life, including physical and mental health, as well as social and interpersonal relationships.
- Specific screening tools are available for AUD including the CAGE and AUDIT questionnaires and the MAST-G and SMAST-G which have been developed specifically for older adults.
- There are significant gaps in research concerning the 3 FDA-approved pharmacologic treatment options for alcohol use disorder in older adults. Nonpharmacological options are promising.

INTRODUCTION

Chronic conditions such as heart disease, arthritis, and diabetes have increased with the growth of the older adult population.[1] Historically, there has been one chronic condition that declined with increasing age, substance use. However, there is a particularity about baby boomers that was not observed in previously aging populations such as their high use of illicit substances in earlier life.[2] Additionally, it has been observed that substance use, including alcohol, remains high as this population

[a] Department of Psychiatry and Behavioral Neuroscience, Division of Geriatric Psychiatry, St. Louis University School of Medicine, 1438 South Grand Boulevard, St Louis, MO 63104, US; [b] Department of Psychiatry and Behavioral Neuroscience, Division of Geriatric Psychiatry, St. Louis University School of Medicine, 1438 South Grand Boulevard, St Louis, MO 63104, US; [c] Saint Louis University School of Medicine, St. Louis University, 1438 South Grand Boulevard, St Louis, MO 63104, US; [d] Saint Louis University School of Medicine, St. Louis University, 1438 South Grand Boulevard, St Louis, MO 63104, US; [e] Department of Psychiatry and Behavioral Neuroscience, Division of Geriatric Psychiatry, St. Louis University School of Medicine, 1438 South Grand Boulevard, St Louis, MO 63104, USA
* Corresponding author.
E-mail address: gabriela.fenollalmaldonado@health.slu.edu

Clin Geriatr Med 38 (2022) 1–22
https://doi.org/10.1016/j.cger.2021.07.006
0749-0690/22/© 2021 Elsevier Inc. All rights reserved.

transitions into older adulthood, thus making substance use in the elderly one of the fastest growing health problems in the United States (US).[3]

NATURE OF THE PROBLEM AND IMPORTANT DEFINITIONS

There are several theories that may explain the emergence or continuation of substance use disorders in later life. These include increasing older adult populations secondary to increased life expectancy which allows populations to use substances for longer, and as previously noted, it may be secondary to attitudes surrounding drug use, which are unique to the "baby boomers."[4]

In this review, we will be concentrating specifically on alcohol use disorder (AUD), its characterization, effects on health, and treatment. AUD is a disorder with biopsychosocial influences as it adversely affects health, increases the likelihood of psychiatric comorbidities which may increase mortality, and adversely affects family relationships.[5] Thus, because of older adults' health vulnerability, the National Institute of Alcohol Abuse and Alcoholism (NIAAA) recommends not drinking more than one drink per day in women and no more than two per day for men [for older adults aged 65+ years]. It is important to define that one drink is the equivalent of 1 to 1.5 ounces (28 g) of hard liquor.[6]

As defined by the NIAAA, AUD in older adults constitutes an impaired ability to stop or control alcohol use despite adverse health, occupational, or social consequences.[6] This is differentiated from binge alcohol use which is characterized by a pattern of drinking that brings blood alcohol concentrations to 0.08 g/dL, which typically occurs after drinking about 4 drinks in women and 5 in men in a 2-hour period (this must happen on at least 1 day of the month). Moreover, heavy alcohol use is defined as binge drinking that has occurred for 5 or more days in the previous month.[7]

Recent epidemiological studies relative to alcohol use from the 2019 National Survey on Drug Use and Health (NSDUH) reported that the lifetime prevalence of alcohol use in adults aged 65 years or older was 81.9%, with the yearly prevalence of use being 56.1%. Additionally, the percentage of binge alcohol use in older adults was 10.7% and in heavy alcohol use, it was 2.7%. These estimates, although representing a slight decline from the 2014 NSDUH (yearly prevalence of use 62.1%), still encompass a high number of older adults with AUD.[7–10]

According to the NIAAA in the US, alcohol contributes to approximately 18.5% of emergency department visits as well as to 22.1% of overdose deaths related to prescription opioids.[10] Furthermore, there are an estimated 95,000 people (68,000 men and 27,000 women) who die annually from alcohol-related causes, which makes alcohol the third-leading preventable cause of death in the US.[11] Many of these deaths are considered to be attributable to alcohol because its use leads to chronic conditions, such as alcohol-associated liver disease, stroke and heart disease, cirrhosis (unspecified), upper digestive tract cancers, liver cancer, cardiac dysrhythmias, AUD, breast cancer, and hypertension. In the US, in 2020, the economic burden of alcohol misuse cost 249 billion dollars related to health care, crime, and lost work productivity.[12] **(Fig. 1)**. Three-quarters of the total costs of alcohol misuse are associated with binge drinking, including resources, admissions, emergency department visits, and doctor visits.[11]

According to Reczek and colleagues, "heavy alcohol use is strongly associated with (re)marriage and divorce and has significant effects on health in mid to late life."[13] Additionally, alcohol use may increase after divorce secondary to increased levels of stress and emotional turmoil related to the divorce. Furthermore, alcohol use may be most extreme during the transition of divorce, especially in older ages, when the

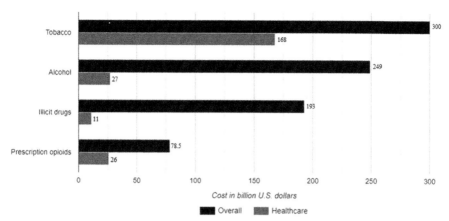

Fig. 1. Costs due to abuse of tobacco, alcohol, illicit drugs, and prescription opioids in the United States as of 2020. (*Data from* Elflein J. Tobacco, alcohol, and illicit drugs abuse costs in the U.S. 2020. Statista. https://www.statista.com/statistics/367863/tobacco-alcohol-and-illicit-drugs-abuse-costs-in-the-us/. Published October 12, 2020. Accessed May 13, 2021.)

loss of marital resources, as well as increased amounts of stress, is most severe.[13] It is difficult to find data specific to the elder population owing to this population being either understudied or underreported; however, the World Health Organization (WHO) reported that the age range with the highest percentage of total deaths attributable to alcohol was between ages 60 and 64 years, with a rate of 17%.[14]

The Diagnostic and Statistical Manual of Mental Disorders of the American Psychiatric Association - 5th Edition (DSM-5) characterizes AUD as a maladaptive pattern of alcohol use that leads to significant impairment or distress in a 12-month period, with specific diagnostic criteria to be met that will be further explained in our article. Furthermore, it is important to note that it can range from mild to severe.[15] Increased or excessive alcohol use may lead to intoxication and withdrawal, which at times may be life-threatening. Intoxication is characterized by clinically problematic behavioral and psychological changes, accompanied by impaired gait, coordination, speech, and attention, which may lead to stupor or coma.[16] Moreover, the typical symptoms for alcohol withdrawal are usually experienced in stages. The first stage starts a few hours after substance abstinence (6–12 hours), and withdrawal symptoms are classified as mild. These may include autonomic instability (changes in blood pressure, heart rate, or breathing rate), tremors, nausea, or vomiting. The second stage of withdrawal usually begins after 12 hours and is characterized by transient alterations of perception, such as visual, auditory, or tactile hallucinations. The third stage occurs 24 to 48 hours after alcohol cessation, and patients may experience tonic-clonic seizures, usually with a brief or no postictal period. Lastly, delirium tremens, which usually can be experienced from 48 to 72 hours, are characterized by rapid fluctuations of perception and consciousness, accompanied by autonomic instability and agitation, which may be life-threatening.[16] Thus, it is important to recognize and treat alcohol withdrawal in its early stages before symptoms become life-threatening. The most effective way to monitor withdrawal symptoms is using the Clinical Institute Withdrawal Assessment for Alcohol (CIWA-Ar) scoring system. The CIWA-Ar is an objective scale that aids in measuring withdrawal severity and comprises a 10-category scale from 0 to 7 (**Table 1**). The maximum score is 67, with 10 to 15 indicating mild withdrawal, 16 to 20 indicating moderate withdrawal, and greater than 20 indicating severe withdrawal. However, it has been suggested that the cutoff for severity may

Table 1
CIWA-Ar scale

Nausea and Vomiting	Headache
0: No nausea/vomiting	0: Not present
1	1: Very mild
2	2: Mild
3	3: Moderate
4: Intermittent nausea with dry heaves	4: Moderately severe
5	5: Severe
6	6: Very severe
7: Constant nausea, vomiting	7: Extremely severe
Auditory Disturbances	Paroxysmal Sweats
0: Not present	0: Not present
1: Very mild harshness	1: Barely perceptible
2: Mild harshness	2
3: Moderate harshness	3
4: Moderately severe	4: Sweat on forehead
5: Severe	5
6: Extremely severe	6
7: Continuous hallucinations	7: Drenching sweat
Anxiety	Visual Disturbances
0: Not present	0: Not present
1	1: Very mild photosensitivity
2	2: Mild photosensitivity
3	3: Moderate photosensitivity
4: Moderately anxious	4: Moderately severe visual hallucinations
5	5: Severe visual hallucinations
6	6: Extremely severe visual hallucinations
7: Acute panic	7: Continuous visual hallucinations
Agitation	Tactile Disturbances
0: Normal	0: Not present
1: Somewhat more than normal	1: Very mild paresthesias
2	2: Mild paresthesias
3	3: Moderate paresthesias
4: Moderately fidgety	4: Moderately severe hallucinations
5	5: Severe hallucinations
6	6: Extremely severe hallucinations
7: Pacing or thrashing during the interview	7: Continuous hallucinations
Tremor	Orientation and clouding sensorium
0: None	0: Normal, can do serial additions
1: Not visible, felt at fingertips	1: Cannot do serial additions
2	2: Disoriented to date for no more than 2 calendar days
3	3: Disoriented to date for more than 2 calendar days
4: Moderate when hands extended	4: Disoriented for place or patient
5	
6	
7: Severe, even when not extended	

Data from Jesse, S., Bråthen, G., Ferrara, M., Keindl, M., Ben-Menachem, E., Tanasescu, R., ... & Ludolph, A. C. (2017). Alcohol withdrawal syndrome: mechanisms, manifestations, and management. Acta Neurologica Scandinavica, 135(1), 4-16.

be lower in elderly patients because of them not showing withdrawal signs the same way and higher possibility of confusion or inability to communicate which may lead to underreporting of symptoms.[17]

Other complications following alcohol withdrawal are Wernicke encephalopathy and the risk of developing Korsakoff's syndrome in the long run. Wernicke's is an acute neurologic condition characterized by a triad of nystagmus, ataxia, and confusion secondary to thiamine deficiency. Moreover, Korsakoff's syndrome involves the progression of the disease and permanent damage to the brain thalamus and hypothalamus.[16] These are particularly relevant on the differential for older adults presenting for delirium or dementia.

DIAGNOSIS OF ALCOHOL USE DISORDER

When diagnosing AUD, we must keep the DSM-5 Diagnostic criteria in mind as the various screening tools for AUD that were developed for older adults were modeled after these criteria. The DSM-5 characteristics of the disorder were defined into 11 criteria.[15] Eight of these 11 criteria relate to a dependence on alcohol: the development of tolerance, having withdrawal effects, desire/unsuccessful efforts to reduce drinking, drinking more than intended/more often, having cravings, spending significant time drinking/recovering from drinking, social/recreational/occupational giving up activities because of alcohol use, or continued drinking despite it causing or exacerbating physical or psychological problems.[15] The other three criteria relate to alcohol abuse, which include failure to fulfill obligations because of alcohol use, continued drinking even in situations where it may be physically hazardous (such as driving), and continued drinking despite harm to relationships with others.[15] For the DSM-5 diagnosis of AUD, two criteria from the total detailed are required to be present in an individual for at least 12 months.[15] AUD is also described in terms of severity: as mild with two or three criteria, moderate with four to five criteria, or severe with six or more criteria met. The caveat with older adults is that screening for these criteria is often missed in the office setting. Explanations for this phenomenon include the need to speed through the visit or that the elderly may be more reticent to discuss their alcohol use. In an effort to combat this, screening tools specific for the elderly have been developed to help identify individuals who may qualify for the diagnosis of AUD.

SCREENING TOOLS
Michigan Alcohol Screening Test-Geriatric Version

One screening tool designed specifically for older adults is the Michigan Alcohol Screening Test-Geriatric Version (MAST-G), which has been adapted from the original Michigan Alcohol Screening Test and tailored to an older adult population. This 24-item questionnaire uses only yes and no answers which may be easier for older adults with possible cognitive impairment. The test also addresses key features of AUD which may be present in older individuals such as the complications of alcohol use. For example, "After a few drinks, have you sometimes not eaten or been able to skip a meal because you didn't feel hungry[18]?" In the 24-item version, 5 or more yes responses indicate a problematic relationship with alcohol may be present, and in the condensed 10-question Short Michigan Alcohol Screening Test-Geriatric Version (SMAT-G), 2 yes responses are required for the indication of AUD.[18] Both versions of this questionnaire have been shown to have comparable sensitivities in detecting hazardous drinking habits in the elderly, .86 for MAST-G and .75 for SMAT-G, and have detected hazardous drinking in geriatric patients not identified by the CAGE Alcohol Questionaire (CAGE) questionnaire, a short screening tool described later in discussion.[19–21]

CAGE Alcohol Questionnaire and Alcohol Use Disorders Identification Test

Although not specific for the elderly, the CAGE questionnaire and the Alcohol Use Disorders Identification Test (AUDIT) screening tools offer a rapid means of screening with each only taking less than 5 minutes to complete and could even be quickly filled out by patients before a visit.[22] With the CAGE questionnaire, patients are asked 4 questions noted in **Table 1** with regards to cutting down, annoyance at criticism of drinking habits, guilt with drinking, and eye-opener use.[6] With this method, usually 2 or more yes responses indicate that a diagnosis of AUD should be explored by the provider.[23] The AUDIT screening tool has both a long and short form, consisting of 10 and 3 questions, respectively, with similar questions to the CAGE. However, the AUDIT also asks about the number of standard drinks an individual typically consumes, how often they drink, and specifically how often they have more than 6 drinks on 1 occasion.[24–26] When examining sensitivity in geriatric patients, the AUDIT was seen to be superior in identifying geriatric patients with alcohol abuse, whereas the CAGE has been shown to be more sensitive in identifying older adults with dependence symptoms.[27] **Table 2** details the commonly used screening tools for AUD in older adults.

DISCUSSION
Psychological Impact of Alcohol Use Disorder on Patients

Depression/link to suicide

Some of the most common psychiatric illnesses observed in the older adult population are depressive disorders, with a prevalence of 10% to 20%, as per the WHO; however, depression among older adults is often underrecognized and underdiagnosed.[14] It is important to note that older adult patients with depression may present with alcohol use or dependence arising for the first time later in their lives.[14] Thorough anamnesis from the patient and collateral is important to establish this connection and to provide clarity. The elder population with depression is at a higher risk for completed suicide or self-harm than their younger counterparts as depression is the most common suicide risk factor in older adults.[28] Thus, each patient must be thoroughly screened and evaluated for suicidal thoughts and/or behaviors.[28] Risk factors for suicide among the elderly who suffer from depression include older age and male gender, severe anxiety, severe depression, domiciled alone, panic attacks, bereavement (more so in men), physical pain, previous suicide attempt(s), and comorbid alcohol/drug use. In a study by Carvalho and colleagues, the Dahlgren–Whitehead rainbow model was used to determine the elderly's risk of becoming ill, their ability to prevent illness, or their access to effective treatments based on economic, environmental, and social inequalities. It was determined that alcohol consumption is one of the main risk factors to demonstrate influence on morbidity and mortality in the elder population.[29,30] "These harmful habits are intensified by the vulnerability of the elderly facing aging changes, loss of friends and family, loneliness, social isolation, and financial difficulties."[29] Also, in case studies, significant associations were found between alcohol and an increase of psychotropic drug use in the elderly. Alcohol was found to be an intermediate determinant among suicide risk factors and as a modifiable factor subject to intervention.[29,30]

"Chicken or the egg" issue

When discussing depression and the use of alcohol, the question arises, what is the primary cause, alcohol use or depression—a "chicken or egg" issue, also known as a causality dilemma. Do older adults use alcohol to cope with mental health concerns,

Table 2
AUD geriatric screening tools

Screening Tool Name	Questions Asked	Scoring Rubric
MAST-G[14]	1. After drinking have you ever noticed an increase in your heart rate or beating in your chest? 2. When talking with others do you ever underestimate how much you actually drink? 3. Does alcohol make you sleepy so that you often fall asleep in your chair? 4. After a few drinks, have you sometimes not eaten, or skipped a meal because you didn't feel hungry? 5. Does having a few drinks help decrease your shakiness or tremors? 6. Does alcohol sometimes make it hard for you to remember parts of the day or night? 7. Do you have rules for yourself that you won't drink before a certain time of the day? 8. Have you lost interest in hobbies or activities that you used to enjoy? 9. When you wake up in the morning do you ever have trouble remembering parts of the night before? 10. Does a drink help you sleep? 11. Do you hide your alcohol bottles from family members? 12. After a social gathering have you ever felt embarrassed because you drank too much? 13. Have you ever been concerned that drinking might be harmful to your health? 14. Do you like to end the evening with a night cap? 15. Did you find that your drinking increased after someone close to you died? 16. In general, would you prefer to have a few drinks at home rather than go out to social events? 17. Are you drinking more now than in the past? 18. Do you usually take a drink to relax or calm your nerves?	≥5 yes responses indicative of problems with alcohol

(continued on next page)

Table 2 (continued)		
Screening Tool Name	**Questions Asked**	**Scoring Rubric**
	19. Do you drink to take your mind off of your problems?	
	20. Have you ever increased your drinking after experiencing a loss in your life?	
	21. Do you sometimes drive when you have had too much to drink?	
	22. Has a doctor or nurse ever said they were worried or concerned about your drinking?	
	23. Have you ever made rules to manage your drinking?	
	24. When you feel lonely does having a drink help?	
SMAST-G[14]	1. When talking with others, do you ever underestimate how much you drink?	≥2 responses indicative of problems with alcohol
	2. After a few drinks, have you sometimes not eaten or been able to skip a meal because you didn't feel hungry?	
	3. Does having a few drinks help decrease your shakiness or tremors?	
	4. Does alcohol sometimes make it hard for you to remember parts of the day or night?	
	5. Do you usually take a drink to calm your nerves?	
	6. Do you drink to take your mind off your problems?	
	7. Have you ever increased your drinking after experiencing a loss in your life?	
	8. Has a doctor or nurse ever said they were worried or concerned about your drinking?	
	9. Have you ever made rules to manage your drinking?	
	10. When you feel lonely, does having a drink help?	
CAGE[22]	1. Have you ever felt you needed to cut down on your drinking?	≥2 responses indicative of problems with alcohol
	2. Have people annoyed you by criticizing your drinking?	
	3. Have you ever felt guilty about drinking?	
	4. Have you ever felt you needed a drink first thing in the morning (eye-opener) to steady your nerves or to get rid of a hangover?	
		(continued on next page)

Table 2 (continued)		
Screening Tool Name	**Questions Asked**	**Scoring Rubric**

AUDIT[19]	1. How often do you have a drink containing alcohol?
	  0 = Never (Skip to Questions 9–10)
	  1 = Monthly or less 2 = 2 to 4 times a month
	  3 = 2 to 3 times a week
	  4 = 4 or more times a week
	2. How many drinks containing alcohol do you have on a typical day when you are drinking?
	  0 = 1 or 2
	  1 = 3 or 4
	  2 = 5 or 6
	  3 = 7, 8, or 9
	  4 = 10 or more
	3. How often do you have six or more drinks on one occasion?
	  0 = Never
	  1 = Less than monthly
	  2 = Monthly
	  3 = Weekly
	  4 = Daily or almost daily
	4. How often during the last year have you found that you were not able to stop drinking once you had started?
	  0 = Never
	  1 = Less than monthly
	  2 = Monthly
	  3 = Weekly
	  4 = Daily or almost daily
	5. How often during the last year have you failed to do what was normally expected from you because of drinking?
	  0 = Never
	  1 = Less than monthly
	  2 = Monthly
	  3 = Weekly
	  4 = Daily or almost daily
	6. How often during the last year have you been unable to remember what happened the night before because you had been drinking?
	  0 = Never
	  1 = Less than monthly
	  2 = Monthly
	  3 = Weekly
	  4 = Daily or almost daily
		≥ 8 indicates hazardous drinking.
		≥ 15 score indicative of a problem with alcohol in men
		≥ 13 score indicative of a problem with alcohol in women

(continued on next page)

Table 2
(continued)

Screening Tool Name	Questions Asked	Scoring Rubric
	7. How often during the last year have you needed an alcoholic drink first thing in the morning to get yourself going after a night of heavy drinking? 0 = Never 1 = Less than monthly 2 = Monthly 3 = Weekly 4 = Daily or almost daily 8. How often during the last year have you had a feeling of guilt or remorse after drinking? 0 = Never 1 = Less than monthly 2 = Monthly 3 = Weekly 4 = Daily or almost daily 9. Have you or someone else been injured as a result of your drinking? 0 = No 2 = Yes, but not in the last year 4 = Yes, during the last year 10. Has a relative, friend, doctor, or another health professional expressed concern about your drinking or suggested you cut down? 0 = No 2 = Yes, but not in the last year 4 = Yes, during the last year	
Short-form AUDIT[17,18]	1. How often do you have a drink containing alcohol? 0 = never 1 = monthly or less 2 = 2–4 times a month 3 = 2–3 times a week 4 = 4 or more times a week 2. How many standard drinks containing alcohol do you have on a typical day when drinking? 0 = 1 or 2 1 = 3 or 4 2 = 5 or 6 3 = 7 to 9 4 = 10 or more 3. How often do you have ≥ 6 drinks on 1 occasion? 0 = never 1 = less than monthly 2 = monthly 3 = weekly 4 = daily or almost daily	≥ 4 score indicative of problem with alcohol in men ≥ 3 score indicative of a problem with alcohol in women

or has chronic drinking been the driving factor in the development of their mental health conditions? It is often difficult to make this distinction, especially when following the criteria for depression AUD according to the DSM-5. Although alcohol sometimes plays the role of a coping strategy for mental distress, other times, alcohol use itself causes mental distress after intake. However, in other instances, alcohol use can relieve mental distress in the short term but exacerbate it in the long term. The effects of alcohol intake on depressive disorders and episodes in the elderly are under-studied. Despite this fact, alcohol consumption is increasing in many countries and excessive intake is particularly climbing in the elderly, which has been shown to have an association with depressive episodes. A study by Keyes and colleagues across 19 countries found that alcohol consumption was differentially associated with the incidence of depressive episodes across different drinking criteria; they observed that the rates of increased depressive episodes were highest among high- and low-alcohol consumers, those being long-term alcohol abstainers, and heavy drinkers.[30] It is notable that, after drinking, women were the most likely to develop a depressive episode when compared with men.[30]

Impact of Alcohol Use Disorder on Organ Systems

Digestive diseases

Alcohol is a causal factor implicated in a variety of medical disorders and is the most used, and abused, drug around the world.[31] Consequences of excessive and pro-longed alcohol consumption include cirrhosis; gastrointestinal (GI) hemorrhage; various malignancies such as oral, pharyngeal/laryngeal, colorectal, hepatic, and esophageal cancers; vitamin deficiencies, especially thiamine; and pancreatitis. Cirrhosis as well as acute and chronic pancreatitis are proportionally linked to alcohol consumption; the higher the alcohol consumption, the higher the risk of developing these diseases.[31] After hepatitis C virus–related chronic liver disease, alcohol repre-sents the most common cause of chronic liver disease.[32] In the US alone, it contrib-utes to approximately 20% to 25% of cases of cirrhosis and roughly 50% of all hospital admissions among patients with cirrhosis.[33] Alcohol and its metabolites also directly injure pancreatic cells through necrosis–fibrosis, a sequence that leads to eventual atrophy and scarring of the pancreas—morphological hallmarks of alco-holic chronic pancreatitis.[33] According to the data collected by Metha and colleagues, acute pancreatitis is the most common GI cause of hospitalization in the US, with approximately 30% of cases being alcohol-induced.[32,34] GI hemorrhage is another possible complication impacted by alcohol abuse. GI hemorrhage represents a frequent cause of intensive care unit admission and has a significant annual incident of approximately 100 cases per 100,000 in the US.[34] Of the most common causes of GI bleeds, mucosal erosions, peptic ulcer disease, and esophageal varices made up more than 80% of the cases, all of which were associated with alcohol abuse.[35]

In 2016, there were an estimated 637,000 digestive disease deaths and 23.3 million digestive disease disabilities associated with harmful alcohol consumption; of those, alcohol-attributable liver cirrhosis led to 607,000 deaths and 22.2 million disabilities-adjusted life years (DALYs). Also in 2016, alcohol-attributable pancreatitis led to 30,000 deaths and 1.1 million DALYs.[14] Furthermore, the harmful consumption of alcohol leads to roughly 3.0 million deaths per year while also taking into consideration the estimated benefit from low levels of alcohol use on some diseases in some population groups.[14]

Endocrine diseases

Mounting evidence demonstrates alcohol's negative effects on one of the body's most crucial systems, the endocrine system, which includes the hypothalamus, pituitary gland, adrenal glands, gonads, thyroid, pancreas, hormones, and adipose tissue.[37] Alcohol, in high consumption, may disrupt all of these interconnected systems leading to hormonal disturbances which may result in various conditions or disorders, such as thyroid issues, immune abnormalities, stress intolerance, psychological and behavioral disorders, and reproductive dysfunction.[37] Diabetes mellitus is a significant and increasing cause of death and morbidity around the world, both directly and indirectly, because of its effects on the kidneys and cardiovascular system. There exists a growing consensus that the consumption of alcohol is an influential factor; however, the exact biologic mechanism remains uncertain. There are some factors that might explain the association including changes in levels of alcohol metabolites, increases in insulin sensitivity after moderate alcohol consumption, increases in HDL cholesterol concentrations, or through the anti-inflammatory effect of alcohol.[38,39] Low to moderate alcohol consumption has been found to reduce the risk of diabetes mellitus because of its improvement in insulin sensitivity.[38] Ley and colleagues report that "based on a meta-analysis, the amounts of alcohol consumption most protective of diabetes were 24 g/d in women and 22 g/d in men, but alcohol became harmful at a consumption level more than 50 g/d in women and 60 g/d in men."[36,38] Prolonged, heavy intake has been observed to disrupt glucose homeostasis, leading to insulin resistance and, eventually, diabetes mellitus.[37,38] Furthermore, the hypothalamic–pituitary–adrenal axis is one of the most sensitive endocrine pathways sensitive to the toxic effects of alcohol consumption. This hormone system is the main control center for stress response and regulates several of the body's physiological processes, including cardiovascular, immune, and metabolic functions; disrupting this pathway may lead to increased disorders of these systems as well.[37]

Peripheral nervous system
When discussing hazardous alcohol consumption, it is also important to note the effects on the peripheral nervous system as well. Alcohol abuse has been associated with a variety of neurologic disorders, including cognitive impairment, cerebellar ataxia, confusion, and peripheral neuropathy.[40,41] It has also been associated with various vitamin deficiencies, including those necessary for proper nerve function, such as vitamins B1 (thiamine), vitamin B6 (pyridoxine), and B12 (cobalamin), the most important of these deficiencies when discussing peripheral neuropathies being vitamin B1.[29,40,41] Prolonged alcohol intake results in thiamine deficiency and can cause peripheral neuropathies which most often manifest as bilateral lower extremity mixed motor and sensory neuropathies, which can present as lower limb weakness with pain, burning sensation, hyperesthesia, and/or numbness.Although older adults are more likely to suffer from diabetic neuropathy, alcohol-related neuropathy is a preventable cause of comorbidity.[42,43]

Cardiovascular
Alcohol also exerts its effects on the cardiovascular and renal systems, contributing to hypertensive disease, cardiomyopathy and heart failure, arrhythmias, as well as hemorrhagic and other nonischemic strokes.[44] Importantly, it is a preventable and modifiable cause of these cardiovascular comorbidities; however, there has been little focus on the effects of alcohol consumption in the older population and while low to moderate intake could be of greatest benefit, abuse could have more severe detrimental effects. When discussing hypertension, the exact mechanism by which alcohol induces increased blood pressure remains unclear. Though there is limited research on the effect of alcohol on hypertension in the geriatric population, there does seem to be a consensus that the association between the two in this population is J-shaped

(semiparabolic).[45] In a study by Jaubert and colleagues, 24 ambulatory and various in-office blood pressure measurements in 533 adults with a mean age of 70 ± 10 years were obtained. After multivariate analysis, the investigators discovered that the average ambulatory diastolic pressure was significantly more elevated in the moderate-to-heavy group (more than a drink/day). Moreover, very light drinks (1 drink per month to 1 drink per week) demonstrated lower daytime blood pressure variability.[44]

Central nervous system

Furthermore, alcohol abuse is also associated with the risk of an increase of lifelong disabling conditions such as dementia. In a multicohort study by Kivimäki and colleagues, 7 cohorts from the United Kingdom, Sweden, France, and Finland including 131,415 adults [mean (SD) age, 43.0 (10.4) years; 80,344 (61.1%) women] were examined.[45] At baseline (1986–2012), participants were between ages 18 and 77 years, reported alcohol use, and were not diagnosed with dementia. Dementia was then examined during an average follow-up of 14.4 years (range, 12.3–30.1). A 1.2-fold excess risk of dementia was demonstrated to be associated with moderate versus heavy alcohol abuse. Also, individuals who reported having an episode of losing consciousness because of alcohol consumption, regardless of overall weekly use, had a 2-fold increased risk of dementia compared with those who did not lose consciousness and were moderate drinkers. After adjusting for possible confounders, the hazard ratio (HR) was 1.16 [95% confidence interval (CI), 0.97–1.37] for consuming more than 14 versus 1 to 14 units of alcohol weekly and 1.22 (95% CI, 1.01–1.48) for more than 21 versus 1 to 21 U weekly. The findings thus suggest an association between alcohol use and the development of dementia, especially in individuals with alcohol-induced loss of consciousness.[45] Koch and colleagues conducted a cohort study of 3021 participants of age 72 years and older and reported "among participants without mild cognitive impairment (MCI) at baseline, daily low-quantity drinking was associated with lower dementia risk than infrequent higher-quantity drinking. Among participants with MCI, consumers of more than 14.0 drinks per week had the most severe cognitive decline than consumers of less than 1.0 drink per week."[46] These results suggest that clinicians and physicians who are involved in the care of geriatric patients should carefully assess and address the full parameters of their patients' drinking patterns, behavior, and cognition when providing support and guidance about their alcohol consumption.

Falls/fractures

Alcohol also plays a role as an important risk factor in different types of injury, such as balance and fall injuries. These are among the top 4 causes of injury death secondary to alcohol consumption, behind road injuries, self-harm, and interpersonal violence.[14] Older adults are at an increased risk for low bone mass or osteoporosis which increases the likelihood of falls and fractures.[47] Additionally, falls and deaths increase with age, but modifiable factors which have been identified and can be addressed exist, including medication and substance use; having a history of alcoholism has been shown to be significantly associated with fall-related injuries.[47] As previously discussed, alcohol is a known cause of certain vitamin deficiencies which may lead to peripheral neuropathies, cognitive impairment, ataxia, and other concerns for balance which could all potentially lead to increasing concerns for falls.[42,43] Being a modifiable risk factor, and considering the increased risk of falls with increasing age, alcohol abuse should be addressed to minimize this risk.

Treatment options for acute intoxication/withdrawal

Benzodiazepines are generally used with caution or not at all in the geriatric population. However, they continue to be the mainstay of treatment for alcohol withdrawal symptoms to help prevent seizures and delirium tremens.[48] The American Society of Addiction Medicine (ASAM) clinical practice guidelines recommend carbamazepine, gabapentin, or phenobarbital for patients with a contraindication to the first-line treatment of benzodiazepines.[49] In older adults, both chlordiazepoxide and diazepam should be avoided because of their extensive liver metabolism and long half-life. Short-acting benzodiazepines such as lorazepam and oxazepam are recommended for those with liver dysfunction.[48] Although limited studies are available on the management of alcohol withdrawal syndrome in older adults, one retrospective health record review set out to evaluate a symptom-triggered protocol approach in patients 70 years and older. The study found that a symptom-triggered protocol approach significantly reduced the duration of treatment as well as cumulative benzodiazepine dose in comparison with a physician-customized management without a protocol.[50]

Treatment Options for Alcohol Use Disorder

Nonpharmacologic options

Adaptive interventions. A recent study assessed adaptive interventions for the treatment of AUD in patients aged 18 to 75 years, with a mean age of 51 years. These included brief advice (BA), motivational interviewing (MI), and behavioral self-control therapy (BSCT). Patients receiving any behavioral self-control therapy had the greatest reductions in drinking. Those who did not initially respond to BA received MI or MI plus BSCT also showed a reduction in alcohol use. For all interventions, prolonged treatment showed improved outcomes.[51]

Cognitive behavioral therapy. Although the need for Cognitive behavioral therapy (CBT) to be effective requires a highly motivated and supported individual, it has been shown to be more effective than no therapy for AUD.[11] One older study examined veterans aged 53 to 82 years who completed an age-specific cognitive behavioral treatment program titled The Geriatric Evaluation Team: Substance Misuse/Abuse Recognition and Treatment (GET SMART).[53] At a 6-month follow-up, 55% of participants who completed at least 13 of 16 GET SMART sessions were significantly more likely to remain abstinent from alcohol than those who did not ($P<.001$).[53] Of note, 35% of participants had previously been treated for alcohol and more than half had previously attended Alcoholics Anonymous (AA) meetings.

Self-Help Groups for AUD include AA, Rational Recovery, and Self-Management and Recovery Training. AA incorporates a 12-step approach. Members provide peer-to-peer support, have sponsors, and may attend a variety of meetings. A recent Cochrane review published in March 2020 evaluated 27 studies that compared AA and similar Twelve Step Facilitation (TSF) programs with other forms of therapy such as CBT. The review concluded that AA/TSF interventions are more effective than other established treatments for increasing abstinence and produce substantial health care cost benefits for those with AUD.[54] Of note, the average age of participants ranged from 34 to 51 years. One study compared 5-year alcohol and drug treatment outcomes of older adults aged 55 to 77 years versus middle-aged and younger adults, aged 40 to 55 years and 18 to 39 years, respectively. The study found that older adults have longer retention in treatment and are less likely to have people in their lives encouraging alcohol or drug use than younger adults. The same study examined ways in which older age contributes to better treatment outcomes and suggested that smaller AA groups or groups focusing specifically on older adult issues may benefit this population.[55]

Pharmacologic treatment options for alcohol use disorder
Currently, there are 3 Food and Drug Administration (FDA)–approved pharmacologic options for the treatment of AUD in the US, including naltrexone, acamprosate, and disulfiram. The efficacy of each is based on strict medication adherence. There is some evidence supporting the off-label use of topiramate, gabapentin, and varenicline in the treatment of AUD. However, the efficacy and safety of these options for older adults are limited.

Naltrexone is a mu-opioid antagonist that works to alter the euphoric effects of alcohol use. It promotes abstinence, reduces heavy drinking and, for some, curbs cravings. Studies regarding the efficacy of naltrexone specifically in older adults for the treatment of AUD are limited. An older, 12-week, double-blind, placebo-controlled study set out to find the efficacy of naltrexone by following 44 Veterans older than 50 years taking 50 mg a day. The study found a significant reduction in a relapse of subjects on naltrexone (50%) who sampled any alcohol during the study versus placebo (100%).[56] In addition, naltrexone was well tolerated among the subjects, with sleep disturbances and anxiety being the most commonly reported. Another study observed treatment response of 50 mg of naltrexone daily in patients aged 55 years and older who met criteria for Major Depressive Disorder (MDD) along with alcohol dependence. All patients were concomitantly taking 100 mg of sertraline daily and receiving weekly psychosocial support. The study observed 42% of subjects had remission of their depression and no alcohol relapses during the trial.[57] However, in the general adult population, naltrexone's efficacy is well studied. The Combined Pharmacotherapies and Behavioral Interventions for Alcohol Dependence (COMBINE), a large randomized controlled trial (RCT) observed patients taking up to 100 mg of naltrexone a day for 16 weeks.[53] In COMBINE, naltrexone reduced the risk of heavy drinking days (HR: 0.72, 97.5% CI, 0.53–0.98, $P = .02$) and had a significantly higher percentage of days abstinent (80.6%) versus placebo (75.1%). A systematic review and meta-analysis calculated the Number Needed to Treat (NNT) to prevent a return to any drinking when using PO naltrexone 50 mg/d for AUD.[58] The calculated NNT is 20 with 95% CI of 11 to 500 and risk difference (RD) of −0.05; 95% CI, −0.10 to −0.002.[58] A long-acting injectable of naltrexone is available as an alternative option for those struggling with adherence to PO. When compared with placebo for 6 months of therapy, a 25% decrease in the rate of heavy drinking days was observed for 380 mg of IM naltrexone ($P = .02$) and a 17% decrease with 190 mg ($P = .07$).[59] More recently, one study looking at older adults ranging in age from 65 to 83 years taking 50 mg of naltrexone for 2 months for severe pruritus showed no serious adverse effects.[60] However, caution should be taken in those with hepatic dysfunction because there have been cases of hepatotoxicity, demonstrating a need for baseline and periodic liver function tests.[52,61,62] In addition, an alternative may be necessary for those who require opioid analgesics because of its antagonistic effects.[53] It can be given orally at a dose of 50 mg per day or intramuscularly at 380 mg every 4 weeks.[63]

Acamprosate, an N-methyl D-Aspartic Acid (NMDA) and Gamma aminobutyric acid (GABA) receptor modulator, is the alternate option for those with contraindications to naltrexone. Although its safety and efficacy have not been studied in those older than 65 years, its low adverse effect profile across populations deems it relatively safe.[64] A Cochrane review of acamprosate (1332 mg/d) versus placebo analyzed 24 RCTs.[65] Acamprosate was found to significantly reduce the risk of any drinking (RR: 0.86, 95% CI: 0.81–0.9) and increase abstinence duration by 11%.[65] The FDA-approved dose is 1998 mg (666 three times a day) daily for sustaining abstinence in those who are abstinent at treatment initiation.[65] Because of renal excretion, caution and dose adjustment should be taken into consideration in those with impaired kidney function.[63] For creatinine clearance between 30 and 50 mL/min, dose should be lowered to 333 mg, three times daily.[64] Because a decline in kidney function is common with aging, renal functions should be monitored regularly. Of note, when compared with naltrexone, meta-analyses found no statistically significant difference for return to any drinking (RD: 0.02; 95% CI, −0.03–0.08).[58]

Disulfiram inhibits the enzyme aldehyde dehydrogenase, causing a buildup of acetaldehyde in blood when consuming alcohol. This leads to nausea, vomiting, and flushing, creating an aversion to alcohol. Because of the strain these side effects may have on the cardiovascular system (hypotension and arrhythmia), it is usually avoided in older adults.[21,48,64] Patients must be abstinent for at least 12 hours before starting disulfiram. The recommended dose is 250 to 500 mg/d.[65]

Few non–FDA-approved medications are beingused for the treatment of AUD. The current APA guidelines, updated in 2018, include topiramate or gabapentin as an option for patients. These are offered for moderate to severe AUD in patients who wish to reduce their consumption or achieve abstinence, have not responded to the FDA-approved treatments, and have no contraindications to these medications.[66,67] Although baclofen, a GABA B agonist, has recently been discussed for its use in AUD, it has not shown superiority versus placebo.[68] Doses up to 1200 mg/d have shown some efficacy versus placebo in AUD, with less heavy drinking days and improved abstinence.[69] Only moderately beneficial and marginally harmful effects have been observed, making it less ideal for patients of any age with AUD.[68,70] Topiramate has been studied at doses of 25 to 300 mg/d titrated over 8 weeks. Although its mechanism of action in AUD remains unknown, patients had fewer drinks per day and more days abstinent than placebo.[71] Nalmefene, a Mu/Delta opioid receptor antagonist, has also been used off-label in the treatment of AUD.[68,72] However, the evidence to support its use remains weak.

It is important to emphasize the efficacy and safety of the FDA-approved pharmacologic treatment options that have yet to be specifically studied in patients aged 65 years or older with AUD.

Natural History of Alcohol Use Disorder

Once one begins to develop AUD, abstinence can become a lifelong battle. As noted previously, untreated AUD can lead to numerous physiological consequences affecting almost any organ system and may lead to social/economic problems. Studies have set out to observe what may influence the rate of alcohol dependence in adulthood and later life and its effects on the body as one ages.

About 24% of people remain abstinent within the year after treatment of AUD, and 10% are able to remain asymptomatic with moderate drinking.[71] Relapse is complex and influenced by biopsychosocial factors; however, attempts at understanding its causes have been made. One study found that both age and severity of alcohol withdrawal symptoms during hospitalization play a role. A recent prospective study following up 158 alcohol-dependent patients aged 21 to 60 years observed increased odds of relapse; the older a patient was (OR 0.975, $P = .030$), the higher their CIWA-Ar was (CIWA for Alcohol revised, a shortened version of the CIWA), although hospitalized (OR 1.126, $P = .010$).[73] In addition, relapse rates have been shown to be higher in those who report impaired control over [alcohol] use (27.2%), having cravings (22.6%), and continued use despite social or interpersonal problems (21%).[73] However, as more time passes since remission, the observed relapse rate decreases to 12% after 20 years.[74]

Influences on the chronicity of alcohol abuse have been found to be associated with age at first use, gender, and ethnicity.[75,76] One longitudinal study following up 808 participants found that drinking regularly before the age of 21 years had a greater odds of lifetime alcohol dependence (OR: 1.71, *P*<.05). In addition, the earlier the alcohol use is initiated, the greater the rate of alcohol dependence is. Those who initiated use before the age of 11 years had a rate of alcohol dependence 1.62 times greater than those who delayed initiating until 15 to 17 years old (*P*<.01) and 3.67 times greater than those starting at the age of 18 to 20 years (*P*<.05).[77] The same study showed that men are more likely to have lifetime alcohol misuse than women (OR: 2.54, *P*<.01).[75] As abstinence from alcohol remains difficult to obtain, understanding that age, gender, and ethnicity play role in its misuse may be of great importance in screening for and treating AUD.

Alcohol as a "Gateway" Drug: What the Evidence Shows

The current research is focused on adolescence and excludes the older population. Alcohol as a gateway in older adults is an area of research that has yet to be conducted. Research relative to older adults may or may not parallel adolescents because their explanations for drinking may be drastically different. Although children and adolescents are often influenced by their peers, a systematic review summarized some of the potential facilitators of drinking in older adults as follows. Older adults may begin to use alcohol as a part of their social life, fun, and enjoyment. They also tend to adopt the drinking habits of those close to them who view it as a social norm. Some begin drinking for medicinal purposes such as for heart disease or to relieve physical symptoms. The review also found that older adults tend to drink to deal with life's difficulties such as anxiety; loneliness; loss of partners, family, friends; or loss of physical activity and mobility.[78] As polysubstance abuse continues to be a public health concern, addressing early alcohol use may be essential to reducing its abuse later in life.

FUTURE RESEARCH

With regards to further exploration into AUD in older adults, there seems to be a significant gap in research regarding the treatment of specific subsets of the elderly population. One such group is older adults with multiple comorbidities. Although there are recommendations such as avoidance of disulfiram in older individuals because of possible drug–drug interactions with commonly prescribed blood pressure medications, there is a gap in research recommendations on the management of AUD in elderly patients. Complicating issues such as polypharmacy which has become increasingly common in the elderly older than 65 years need to be examined.[22,23] In addition, although there has been evidence that within racial groups there are significant differences in alcohol consumption based on ethnic origins, research has lagged on investigating the access, utilization, effectiveness, and tolerability of current treatments in various racial and ethnic elders.[79] By not addressing each of these subgroups, the complexities of cultural norms surrounding alcohol, beliefs regarding medical treatment, and the ability to access the health care system are being missed.

SUMMARY

Research on hazardous alcohol use specifically in the older adult population is limited; however, long-term adverse effects of prolonged alcohol use are seen in this group. Alcohol use has well-documented adverse effects on individuals and public health. It is imperative to create, support, and enforce efforts to mitigate its harmful use not only in the younger population but also in older adults through alcohol policy as well as other policies and measures that are not enforced or implemented, such as education on consumption, effects, and long-term complications. It is hoped that this project can raise awareness relative to the need to understand alcohol abuse in the older adult population so that its effects and ramifications can be better identified and addressed and proper interventions can be made to reduce the harmful effects of alcohol in this vulnerable population.

CLINICS CARE POINTS

- Although there are currently 3 FDA-approved medications for the treatment of AUD, naltrexone remains the mainstay of treatment because of its side effect profile and efficacy.
- Chronic alcohol use affects multiple organ systems as well as mental health which may be especially important to monitor in older adults because they are at a higher risk for medical comorbidities and completed suicide.
- Screening tools have been developed specifically for AUD in the older adult population including the MAST-G and the shorter SMAST-G questionnaires with comparable sensitivities and specificity for screening for AUD.

DISCLOSURE

The authors have nothing to disclose.

REFERENCES

1. Christensen K, Doblhammer G, Rau R, et al. Ageing populations: the challenges ahead. Lancet (London, England) 2009;374(9696):1196–208.
2. Yarnell S, Li L, MacGrory B, et al. Substance use disorders in later life: a review and synthesis of the literature of an emerging public health concern. Am J Geriatr Psychiatry 2020;28(2):226–36.
3. Colby SL, Ortman JM. The baby boom cohort in the United States: 2012 to 2060. Current population reports. Washington, DC: US Census Bureau; 2014. p. 25–1141.
4. Colliver JD, Compton WM, Gfroerer JC, et al. Projecting drug use among aging baby boomers in 2020. Ann Epidemiol 2006;16:257–65.
5. McGrath A, Crome P, Crome IB. Substance misuse in the older population. Postgrad Med J 2005;81(954):228–31.
6. National Institute of alcohol abuse and alcoholism. Older adults. Bethesda, MD: NIAAA; 2017. Available at: https://www.niaaa.nih.gov/alcohol-health/special-populations-co-occurring- disorders/older-adults.
7. Han BH, Moore AA. Prevention and screening of unhealthy substance use by older adults. Clin Geriatr Med 2018;34(1):117–29.
8. Han BH, Moore AA, Sherman S, et al. Demographic trends of binge alcohol use and alcohol use disorders among older adults in the United States, 2005–2014. Drug and Alcohol Dependence 2016;170:198–207.
9. Substance abuse and mental health services administration. 2019. Available at: https://www.samhsa.gov/data/report/2019-nsduh-detailed-tables. Accessed April 30, 2021.
10. Alcohol facts and statistics. National Institute on Alcohol Abuse and Alcoholism. Available at: https://www.niaaa.nih.gov/publications/brochures-and-fact-sheets/alcohol-facts-and-statist.

11. Magill M, Ray L, Kiluk B, et al. A meta-analysis of cognitive-behavioral therapy for alcohol or other drug use disorders: treatment efficacy by contrast condition. J Consul Clin Psychol 2019;87(12):1093–105.
12. Elflein J. Tobacco, alcohol, and illicit drugs abuse costs in the U.S. 2020. Statista 2020. Available at: https://www.statista.com/statistics/367863/tobacco-alcohol-and-illicit-drugs-abuse-costs-in-the-us/. Accessed May 13, 2021.
13. Reczek C, Pudrovska T, Carr D, et al. Marital histories and heavy alcohol use among older adults [published correction appears in J health soc behav. 2016 Jun;57(2):274]. J Health Soc Behav 2016;57(1):77–96.
14. Global status report on alcohol and health 2018. World Health Organization. Available at: https://apps.who.int/iris/handle/10665/274603. License: CC BY-NC-SA 3.0 IGO. Accessed April 8, 2021.
15. American Psychiatric Association. Diagnostic and statistical manual of mental disorders. 5th edition. Arlington, VA: American Psychiatric Publishing; 2013.
16. Jesse S, Bråthen G, Ferrara M, et al. Alcohol withdrawal syndrome: mechanisms, manifestations, and management. Acta Neurol Scand 2017;135(1):4–16.
17. Identification and management of alcohol abuse and withdrawal in elders. consultant360.com. Available at: https://www.consultant360.com/articles/identification-and-management-alcohol-abuse-and-withdrawal-elders.
18. Blow FC, Brower KJ, Schulenberg JE, et al. The Michigan Alcoholism Screening Test- Geriatric Version (MAST-G): A new elderly-specific screening instrument. Alcohol Clin Exp Res 1992;16:372.
19. Johnson-Greene D, McCaul ME, Roger P. Screening for hazardous drinking using the Michigan alcohol screening test-geriatric version (MAST-G) in elderly persons with acute cerebrovascular accidents. Alcohol Clin Exp Res 2009;33(9):1555–61.
20. Kaufman DW, Kelly JP, Rosenberg L, et al. Recent patterns of medication use in the ambulatory adult population of the United States: the slone Survey. JAMA 2002;287(3):337–44.
21. Kuerbis Alexis, Paul Sacco. A review of existing treatments for substance abuse among the elderly and recommendations for future directions. Subst Abuse 2013; 7. SART.S7865.
22. Moore AA, Seeman T, Morgenstern H, et al. 'Are there differences between older persons who screen positive on the CAGE questionnaire and the short Michigan alcoholism screening test—geriatric version?'. J Am Geriatr Soc 2002;50(5): 858–62.
23. O'Brien CP. The CAGE questionnaire for detection of alcoholism. JAMA 2008; 300(17):2054.
24. Babor TF, Higgins-Biddle JC, Saunders JB, et al. AUDIT: the alcohol use disorders identification test: guidelines for use in primary care. 2nd edition. Geneva (Switzerland): World Health Organization; 2001.
25. Bush K, Kivlahan DR, McDonell MB, et al. The AUDIT alcohol consumption questions (AUDIT-C): an effective brief screening test for problem drinking. Ambulatory Care Quality Improvement Project (ACQUIP). Alcohol Use Disorders Identification Test. Arch Intern Med 1998;158(16):1789–95.
26. Berks J, McCormick R. Screening for alcohol misuse in elderly primary care patients: a systematic literature review. Int Psychogeriatr 2008;20(6):1090–103.
27. Hays RD, Laural H, Gillogly JJ, et al. Response Times for the CAGE, Short-MAST, AUDIT, and JELLINEK alcohol scales. Behav Res Methods Instrum Comput 1993; 25.2:304–7.
28. Avasthi A, Grover S. Clinical practice guidelines for management of depression in elderly. Indian J Psychiatry 2018;60(Suppl 3):S341–62.

29. Carvalho ML, Costa AP, Monteiro CF, et al. Suicide in the elderly: approach to so-cial determinants of health in the Dahlgren and Whitehead model. Rev Bras Enferm 2020;73(suppl 3).

30. Keyes KM, Allel K, Staudinger UM, et al. Alcohol consumption predicts incidence of depressive episodes across 10 years among older adults in 19 countries. Int Rev Neurobiol 2019;148:1–38.

31. Mehta AJ. Alcoholism and critical illness: a review. World J Crit Care Med 2016; 5(1):27–35.

32. Singal AK, Anand BS. Recent trends in the epidemiology of alcoholic liver disease. Clin Liv Dis 2013;2:53–6.

33. Rocco A, Compare D, Angrisani D, et al. Alcoholic disease: liver and beyond. World J Gastroenterol 2014;20(40):14652–9.

34. Peery AF, Dellon ES, Lund J, et al. Burden of gastrointestinal disease in the United States: 2012 update. Gastroenterology 2012;143(5):1179–87.e3.

35. Bang CS, Lee YS, Lee YH, et al. Characteristics of nonvariceal upper gastrointestinal hemorrhage in patients with chronic kidney disease. World J Gastroenterol 2013;19(43):7719–25.

36. Baliunas DO, Taylor BJ, Irving H, et al. Alcohol as a risk factor for type 2 diabetes: a systematic review and meta-analysis. Diabetes Care 2009;32(11):2123–32.

37. Rachdaoui N, Sarkar DK. Pathophysiology of the effects of alcohol abuse on the endocrine system. Alcohol Res 2017;38(2):255–76.

38. Ley SH, Hamdy O, Mohan V, et al. Prevention and management of type 2 diabetes: dietary components and nutritional strategies. Lancet 2014;383(9933): 1999–2007.

39. Hendriks HFJ. Moderate alcohol consumption and insulin sensitivity: observations and possible mechanisms. Ann Epidemiol 2007;17(5). https://doi.org/10.1016/j.annepidem.2007.01.009.

40. Piano MR. Alcohol's effects on the cardiovascular system. Alcohol Res 2017; 38(2):219–41.

41. Kalla A, Figueredo VM. Alcohol and cardiovascular disease in the geriatric population. Clin Cardiol 2017;40(7):444–9.

42. Julian T, Glascow N, Syeed R, et al. Alcohol-related peripheral neuropathy: a systematic review and meta-analysis. J Neurol 2019;266(12):2907–19.

43. Chopra K, Tiwari V. Alcoholic neuropathy: possible mechanisms and future treatment possibilities. Br J Clin Pharmacol 2012;73(3):348–62.

44. Jaubert MP, Jin Z, Russo C, et al. Alcohol consumption and ambulatory blood pressure: a community-based study in an elderly cohort. Am J Hypertens 2014;27(5):688–94.

45. Kivimäki M, Singh-Manoux A, Batty GD, et al. Association of alcohol-induced loss of consciousness and overall alcohol consumption with risk for dementia. JAMA Netw Open 2020;3(9):e2016084.

46. Koch M, Fitzpatrick AL, Rapp SR, et al. Alcohol consumption and risk of dementia and cognitive decline among older adults with or without mild cognitive impairment. JAMA Netw Open 2019;2(9):e1910319.

47. Chen CM, Yoon YH. Usual alcohol consumption and risks for nonfatal fall injuries in the United States: results from the 2004-2013 national health interview Survey. Subst Use Misuse 2017;52(9):1120–32.

48. Le Roux C, Tang Y, Drexler K. Alcohol and opioid use disorder in older adults: neglected and treatable illnesses. Curr Psychiatry Rep 2016;18(9):87.

49. The ASAM clinical practice guideline on alcohol withdrawal management. J Addict Med 2020;14(3S Suppl 1):1–72.

50. Taheri A, Dahri K, Chan P, et al. Evaluation of a symptom-triggered protocol approach to the management of alcohol withdrawal syndrome in older adults. J Am Geriatr Soc 2014;62(8):1551–5.

51. Morgenstern J, Kuerbis A, Shao S, et al. An efficacy trial of adaptive interventions for alcohol use disorder. J Substance Abuse Treat 2021;123:108264.

52. Anton RF, O'Malley SS, Ciraulo DA, et al, COMBINE Study Research Group. Combined pharmacotherapies and behavioral interventions for alcohol dependence: the COMBINE study: a randomized controlled trial. JAMA 2006;295(17):2003–17.

53. Schonfeld L, Dupree LW, Dickson-Euhrmann E, et al. Cognitive-behavioral treatment of older veterans with substance abuse problems. J Geriatr Psychiatry Neurol 2000;13(3):124–9.

54. Kelly JF, Humphreys K, Ferri M. Alcoholics Anonymous and other 12-step programs for alcohol use disorder. Cochrane Database Syst Rev 2020;3(3): CD012880.

55. Satre DD, Mertens JR, Areán PA, et al. Five-year alcohol and drug treatment outcomes of older adults versus middle-aged and younger adults in a managed care program. Addiction 2004;99(10):1286–97.

56. Oslin D, Liberto JG, O'Brien J, et al. Naltrexone as an adjunctive treatment for older patients with alcohol dependence. Am J Geriatr Psychiatry 1997;5(4): 324–32.

57. Oslin DW. Treatment of late-life depression complicated by alcohol dependence. Am J Geriatr Psychiatry 2005;13(6):491–500.

58. Jonas DE, Amick HR, Feltner C, et al. Pharmacotherapy for adults with alcohol use disorders in outpatient settings: a systematic review and meta-analysis. JAMA 2014;311(18):1889–900.

59. Garbutt JC, Kranzler HR, O'Malley SS, et al, Vivitrex Study Group. Efficacy and tolerability of long-acting injectable naltrexone for alcohol dependence: a randomized controlled trial. JAMA 2005;293(13):1617–25.

60. Lee J, Shin JU, Noh S, et al. Clinical efficacy and safety of naltrexone combination therapy in older patients with severe pruritus. Ann Dermatol 2016;28(2):159–63.

61. Singh D, Saadabadi A. Naltrexone. [Updated 2021 Aug 6]. In: StatPearls [Internet]. Treasure Island (FL): StatPearls Publishing; 2021 Jan-. Available from: https://www.ncbi.nlm.nih.gov/books/NBK534811/

62. Kranzler HR, Soyka M. Diagnosis and pharmacotherapy of alcohol use disorder: a review. JAMA 2018;320(8):815–24.

63. Reus VI, Fochtmann LJ, Bukstein O, et al. The American psychiatric association practice guideline for the pharmacological treatment of patients with alcohol use disorder. Am J Psychiatry 2018;175(1):86–90.

64. FDA label acamprosate. Available at: https://www.accessdata.fda.gov/drugsatfda_docs/label/2012/021431s015lbl.pdf.

65. Stokes M, Abdijadid S. Disulfiram. In: StatPearls. Treasure Island (FL): StatPearls Publishing; 2021. Available at: https://www.ncbi.nlm.nih.gov/books/NBK459340/.

66. Guerbis A, Sacco P, Blazer DG, et al. Substance abuse among older adults. Clin Geriatr Med 2014;30(3):629–54.

67. Rösner S, Hackl-Herrwerth A, Leucht S, et al. Acamprosate for alcohol dependence. Cochrane database Syst Rev 2010;(9):CD004332.

68. Minozzi S, Saulle R, Rösner S. Baclofen for alcohol use disorder. Cochrane database Syst Rev 2018;11(11):CD012557.

69. Anton RF, Latham P, Voronin K, et al. Efficacy of gabapentin for the treatment of alcohol use disorder in patients with alcohol withdrawal symptoms: a randomized clinical trial. JAMA Intern Med 2020;180(5):728–36.

70. Bschor T, Henssler J, Müller M, et al. Baclofen for alcohol use disorder-a systematic meta-analysis. Acta Psychiatr Scand 2018;138(3):232–42.
71. Miller WR, Walters ST, Bennett ME. How effective is alcoholism treatment in the United States? J Stud alcohol 2001;62(2):211–20.
72. Miyata H, Takahashi M, Murai Y, et al. Nalmefene in alcohol-dependent patients with a high drinking risk: randomized controlled trial. Psychiatry Clin Neurosci 2019;73(11):697–706.
73. Xhu R, Ni ZJ, Zhang S, et al. [Effect of clinical characteristics on relapse of alcohol dependence: a prospective cohort study]. Beijing Da Xue Xue Bao Yi Xue Ban 2019;51(3):519–24.
74. Tuithof M, ten Have M, van den Brink W, et al. Alcohol consumption and symptoms as predictors for relapse of DSM-5 alcohol use disorder. Drug Alcohol Depend 2014;140:85–91.
75. Guttmannova K, Bailey JA, Hill KG, et al. Sensitive periods for adolescent alcohol use initiation: predicting the lifetime occurrence and chronicity of alcohol problems in adulthood. J Stud Alcohol Drugs 2011;72(2):221–31.
76. Vaeth PA, Wang-Schweig M, Caetano R. Drinking, alcohol use disorder, and treatment access and utilization among U.S. Racial/ethnic groups. Alcohol Clin Exp Res 2017;41(1):6–19.
77. Barrense-Dias, Y., Berchtold, A., Akre, C., & Surís, J. C. (2016). Alcohol misuse and gateway theory: a longitudinal study among adolescents in Switzerland. International journal of adolescent medicine and health, 30(1), /j/ijamh.2018.30.issue-1/ijamh-2016-0004/ijamh-2016-0004.xml.
78. Kelly S, Olanrewaju O, Cowan A, et al. Alcohol and older people: a systematic review of barriers, facilitators and context of drinking in older people and implications for intervention design. PLoS One 2018;13(1):e0191189.
79. Martins de Carvalho L, Wiers CE, Manza P, et al. Effect of alcohol use disorder on cellular aging. Psychopharmacology 2019;236(11):3245–55.

Screening for and Management of Opioid Use Disorder in Older Adults in Primary Care

Rajat Duggirala, MD[a], Sunil Khushalani, MD, DFAPA[b],
Todd Palmer, MD[c], Nicole Brandt, PharmD, MBA, BCGP, BCPP[d,e,f],
Abhilash Desai, MD[g,h],*

KEYWORDS

• Opioid • Older • Elderly • Addiction • Naloxone • Buprenorphine • Methadone
• Naltrexone

KEY POINTS

• Prevention of Opioid use disorder (OUD) is much easier than treatment, best done by trying to avoid the use of opioids for chronic pain, and if prescribed, using the lowest possible dose for the shortest possible duration.

• Routine screening for OUD is recommended for all older adults, especially in primary care as it may result in earlier diagnosis, earlier treatment, and reduced morbidity, mortality, and healthcare costs.

• Suspect OUD in patients with characteristic symptoms and signs, especially if they have risk factors, and provide brief intervention, referral if needed, and treatment if possible.

• Evidence shows that Medications for OUD (MOUDs) are very effective in reducing opioid use and in reducing mortality even when used without psychosocial interventions and should not be withheld in patients who refuse or unable to obtain psychosocial interventions.

• Combination of psychosocial behavioral approaches that are age-sensitive along with MOUD are the treatments of choice.

[a] Saint Louis University, 1438 South Grand Boulevard, St Louis, MO 63104, USA; [b] Kolmac Outpatient Recovery Centers, 3919 National Drive, Suite 300, Burtonsville, MD 20866, USA; [c] Addiction Fellowship, Family Medicine Residency of Idaho, 777 North Raymond Street, Boise, ID 83704, USA; [d] MedStar Center for Successful Aging, 220 Arch St, 12th Floor, Baltimore, MD 21201, USA; [e] University of Maryland School of Pharmacy; [f] The Peter Lamy Center on Drug Therapy and Aging; [g] Department of Psychiatry and Behavioral Sciences, University of Washington School of Medicine, 413 North Allumbaugh Street, Suite#101, Boise, ID 83704, USA; [h] Department of Psychiatry and Behavioral Sciences, University of Washington School of Medicine
* Corresponding author.
E-mail address: dr.abhilashdesai@icloud.com

Clin Geriatr Med 38 (2022) 23–38
https://doi.org/10.1016/j.cger.2021.07.001
0749-0690/22/© 2021 Elsevier Inc. All rights reserved.

INTRODUCTION

Opioid misuse (OM) describes a broad clinical syndrome of using opioids without a prescription or in doses and frequencies greater than prescribed, and for purposes other than its medical use.[1] Data collected from 2006 to 2013 found that 35% of adults older than 50 years reported OM in the past 30 days.[2] OM is often associated with untreated or undertreated pain in older adults and often co-occurs with misuse of other illicit drugs such as marijuana.[3] OM in older adults leads to severe physical and psychiatric morbidity.[4]

Opioid use disorder (OUD) is a clinical diagnosis involving the compulsive use of opioids despite negative consequences and can be thought of as a subset of OM.[1] OUD is a chronic relapsing disease.[5] This diagnosis is becoming more common in older adults.[6,7] With effective treatment of OUD, a cohort of adults with early onset OUD in their twenties and thirties are now aging well into their sixties. Other older adults may also develop OUD later in life in association with prescribed opioids for their chronic pain.[6] Older adults with OUD have higher mortality rates from an accidental overdose, suicide, and violent death compared with their peers without OUD.[8] Additionally, they may be less likely than younger adults to perceive OUD as problematic or to access specialty treatment services.[9]

In general, meeting the unique needs of older adults with OUD will need efforts at all levels of care in health-care systems and range from prevention to intervention and treatment. Reimbursement systems must support a spectrum of approaches that include safe and appropriate opioid prescribing practices, screening for and early detection of OUD, diagnosis, treatment, and ongoing management of patients with OUD.[1] Primary care providers (PCPs) are on the front lines of these efforts illustrated through four patient cases. This clinical review describes the screening, for as well as the management of OM in general, and OUD specifically as applied to primary care.

SCREENING, BRIEF INTERVENTION, AND REFERRAL FOR TREATMENT

Screening, brief intervention and referral for treatment is an approach and a framework designed to systematize and standardize the practice of screening for and addressing substance misuse.[5] While research has primarily identified its effectiveness in hazardous levels of alcohol use, it has applications in identifying OUD and the risk of OUD. Suspect OUD in older adults with characteristic symptoms and or signs, especially if they have risk factors. Please refer to **Table1** and **Box 1**.[1,5,6]

Screening

The Federal Substance Abuse and Mental Health Administration (SAMHSA) recommends at least annual screening for substance misuse, including prescription medications such as opioids.[6] Screening should also occur when major life changes occur for older adults or when family members raise concerns about an older adult's medication or other substance use. **Table 2** lists screening tools that may be used in primary care.[10–15] None of the screening tools listed are as yet validated in older adults. PCPs should communicate the results of a positive screen in a respectful and culturally sensitive manner, emphasizing that an OUD is not a negative judgment but a clinical diagnosis. For patients with a past history of OUD who screen negative, praising them for maintaining abstinence is also important. In high-risk patients (eg, past history of heroin addiction and current mental health challenges), a drug screen (eg, random urine drug screen) is recommended as an additional tool for clinical data.[6] PCPs need to address stigma of addiction at the time of screening. Stigma of

Table 1
Signs and symptoms of OUD, opioid intoxication, and opioid withdrawal

	OUD	Opioid intoxication	Opioid withdrawal
Signs	• Recurrent visits to emergency department for opioid related adverse effects, especially respiratory and or central nervous system depression • Family members noticing frequent drowsiness and or slurred speech in patients on opioids • Use of opioid medications at great frequency or amount than prescribed • Any and all use of illicit opioids • Use of prescription opioids for reasons other than pain management (eg, for its euphoric effects, to "manage" stress, anxiety, depression or dysphoria)	• Bradycardia • Head nodding • Hypokinesis • Hypotension • Hypothermia • Miosis[a] • Respiratory depression • Sedation • Slurred speech • Hypoactive delirium	• Diaphoresis • Hyperreflexia • Hypertension (mild) • Hyperthermia • Tachycardia (mild) • Increased respiratory rate • Lacrimation • Muscle spasms • Mydriasis • Piloerection • Rhinorrhea • Yawning • Agitation • Restlessness • Shivering • Sneezing • Tremor
Symptoms	• Difficulty remembering and thinking • Difficulty staying awake in the daytime • Fatigue • Tiredness	• Analgesia • Calmness • Euphoria	• Abdominal pain and cramps • Leg cramps • Anxiety • Bone and muscle pain • Diarrhea • Anorexia • Nausea/vomiting • Dizziness • Restless leg syndrome

[a] Normal pupillary size does not rule out opioid toxicity.
Data from Olsen Y, Sharfstein JM. The opioid epidemic: what everyone needs to know: Oxford University Press, 20196; and Adults SAAO. Treatment Improvement Protocol (TIP) Series, No. 26. Center for Substance Abuse Treatment. Rockville (MD): Substance Abuse and Mental Health Services Administration (US) 1998.

addiction may make it less likely that older adults will spontaneously share their problems with opioids and accept referrals for treatment.

Brief Intervention and Referral

Education is a key component of brief intervention. Please refer to **Table 3**.[1,5,6] Partnering with family and concerned significant others using a culturally competent approach and assessing beliefs, attitudes, and expectations about OUD treatment is key to successful outcomes in older adults. PCPs should explain to patients and their families that OUD is a medical condition (brain disorder) and not a moral defect. PCPs should explain the serious risks associated with opioid use (**Table 4**), especially risk of overdose death.[1,5,6,16–18] Person-first language should be used, and diligent effort is needed to not use stigmatizing and traumatizing language (**Table 5**).[1,6]

Box 1
Key risk factors for opioid misuse and opioid use disorder in older adults

- Long-term opioid therapy for chronic noncancer pain
- Past history of opioid misuse or opioid use disorder
- Current or past history of other substance misuse and or substance use disorder (eg, benzodiazepines, hypnotics, marijuana)
- Family history of substance use disorders and or psychiatric disorders
- History of psychiatric disorders
- History of adverse childhood experiences or history of severe trauma

Data from Olsen Y, Sharfstein JM. The opioid epidemic: what everyone needs to know: Oxford University Press, 20196; and Joshi P, Shah NK, Kirane HD. Medication-assisted treatment for opioid use disorder in older adults: an emerging role for the geriatric psychiatrist. The American Journal of Geriatric Psychiatry 2019;27(4):455-57.

PCPs should provide education about recognizing opioid overdose and responding to overdose (including effective use of naloxone) to patients, their family, housemates, and friends. PCPs need to help the patient see that accepting treatment is a sign of strength rather than vulnerability.

PCPs should also tackle the ageism (stigma of aging) from the start. It is a myth that older adults do not benefit from OUD treatment. Not only do older adults benefit from medications for opioid use disorder (MOUDs), age-sensitive psychosocial behavioral interventions and family support but they achieve better treatment outcomes than their younger counterparts.[6,19]

PCPs should educate patients and their families that although addiction counseling and mutual-aid support groups are core components of OUD treatment, they are generally not effective by themselves and that OUD treatment should include MOUD.[6] For most patients who screen positive for OUD, PCPs should make a referral

---

Table 2
Screening tools for opioid use disorder in primary care

Situation	Screening tools	Clinical pearls
Routine screening	NIDA quick screen (National Institute for Drug Abuse)	Excellent screening tool for nonopioid drug misuse and use disorder also
Before initiating LTOT[a]	SISAP questionnaire (Screening instrument for Substance Abuse Potential) Opioid risk tool (ORT) DIRE score (Diagnosis, Intractability, Risk and Efficacy)	SISAP and ORT are very brief and easy to use DIRE score is more comprehensive and recommended over SISAP and ORT
In patients on LTOT	SOAPP-R (Screener and Opioid Assessment for Patients with Pain – Revised) COMM (Current Opioid Misuse Measure)	Both, SOAPP-R and COMM are equally good

[a] LTOT: Long-term Opioid Therapy for management of chronic pain.
Data from Refs.[10–15]

Table 3
Education about opioid misuse and opioid use disorder in primary care

Education of patient and family/support persons	Clinical aspects	Team member
OM and OUD are serious chronic brain disorders	Address stigma and shame	Nurse Social worker PCP Psychiatrist[a]
Adverse effects of opioids	Discuss impact of opioids on current meds and medical – psychiatric comorbidity	PCP Pharmacist[a]
Need for routine periodic screening, what screening involves and Importance of honest answers during screening	Involvement of family/support persons is key to accurate early diagnosis	Nurse Social worker PCP
Importance of naloxone in preventing overdose death, and how and when to use it	Explain signs and symptoms of overdose (eg, impaired arousal, respiratory depression [especially respiratory rate <12/min], miosis, cyanosis, hypothermia, seizures, aspiration pneumonia)	Nurse Social worker PCP Pharmacist
Education about local, national and internet-based resources	Mutual aid support groups are a key example	Nurse Social worker Peer support specialist

[a] Psychiatrist and pharmacist may be available virtually as part of collaborative care.
Data from Olsen Y, Sharfstein JM. The opioid epidemic: what everyone needs to know: Oxford University Press, 20196; and Joshi P, Shah NK, Kirane HD. Medication-assisted treatment for opioid use disorder in older adults: an emerging role for the geriatric psychiatrist. The American Journal of Geriatric Psychiatry 2019;27(4):455-57.

to local opioid treatment centers for accurate diagnoses (not just of OUD but also co-occurring substance use disorders [especially alcohol, Benzodiazepines, and marijuana in older adults] and mental health conditions) and comprehensive holistic treatment. SAMHSA-certified programs can exist in intensive outpatient, residential, and hospital settings. Services include treatment of medical opioid withdrawal management, initiation of MOUDs in combination with a variety of psychiatric, behavioral, social, and medical interventions. Older adults do best if opioid treatment centers provide age-appropriate care by providers who are knowledgeable about issues related to aging (6). Motivational interviewing techniques can help PCPs address the patients' ambivalence or reluctance to accept the problem and treatment referral. Providing a wide range of resources (eg, contact information of local addiction treatment centers, local mutual-support group networks, geriatric care managers, reputable online resources, SAMHSA National Helpline [800–622-HELP]) for the patient, as well as for the caregivers (eg, Nar-Anon) is a key component of education and brief intervention. PCPs should also provide emotional support to family and suggest self-care techniques to mitigate burnout. In addition, geriatric psychiatrists can play a key role in prevention and treatment of OUD in older adults by working closely and collaboratively with PCPs as illustrated in care of Ms. T.[20]

Table 4
System-based adverse effects of opioids

System	Adverse effects	Clinical pearls
General	Fatigue Opioid Induced hyperalgesia (OIH) Tolerance Diversion	OIH requires lowering of opioids (increasing opioids worsen pain) Tolerance to analgesic effects may require increase in opioids which in turn may cause more adverse effects
Psychiatric	Addiction (opioid misuse [OM], opioid use disorder [OUD]) Physiologic Dependence Psychological Dependence Withdrawal syndrome Euphoria (immediate effect) Depression (long-term effect) Hallucinations	Individuals with other substance misuse and substance use disorders (current or past) have increased risk of developing OM and OUD Individuals with pre-existing depression and or psychotic disorders are at increased risk of these adverse effects Methadone withdrawal psychosis has been described
Respiratory	Respiratory depression Hypoxia Sleep disordered breathing	Opioids may exacerbate COPD, sleep apnea syndromes, asthma and other pulmonary conditions In palliative and end-of-life settings, opioids may be needed to treat dyspnea
Neurocognitive	Inattention Memory impairment Mental cloudiness Impaired abstract thinking Disorientation Delirium	Individuals with pre-existing mild cognitive impairment or dementia are at higher risk of these adverse effects Individuals on anti-cholinergic medications are at higher risk of these adverse effects Frail older adults are at increased risk of fatigue, falls and injury.
Sleep wake cycle	Daytime sleepiness Nightmares	Individuals with pre-existing OSA and other sleep disorders are at higher risk of these adverse effects
Endocrine	Sexual dysfunction Decreased testosterone levels Amenorrhea Reduced bone mineral density Increased prolactin levels	Individuals with pre-existing osteopenia and osteoporosis may have worsening of their condition with correspondent increased risk of fractures
Urinary	Urinary retention (UR) Urinary incontinence (UI)	Individuals with pre-existing UR and UI are at increased risk of these adverse effects
Neurologic	Incoordination Slurred speech Impaired vision Dizziness Loss of fine motor skills Falls and injury (eg, TBI, fractures)	Individuals with pre-existing neurologic conditions (eg, stroke, TBI, Parkinson's disease) are at increased risk of these adverse effects Opioids can impair driving abilities and this adverse effect needs to be inquired and monitored

(continued on next page)

Table 4 (continued)		
System	**Adverse effects**	**Clinical pearls**
Gastrointestinal	Constipation Intestinal obstruction Anorexia Nausea Vomiting Dry mouth	Individuals with pre-existing gastrointestinal problems (eg, previous abdominal surgeries) are at higher risk of these adverse effects
Dermatologic/Skin changes	Pruritis Rash Diaphoresis	Older adults are often given anticholinergic medications to treat pruritis (eg, hydroxyzine, diphenhydramine) putting them at further risk of cognitive impairment and delirium
Cardiovascular	Hypotension Arrythmias	Methadone prolongs QTc interval more so than other opioids and so should be avoided in older adults with pre-existing cardiac conduction problems. Involvement of a pharmacist is recommended to identify any and all medications that also prolong QTc interval

Data from Refs.[1,6,16–18]

CASE 1: MS. T

Ms. T is a 77-year-old retired nurse currently residing in a nursing home receiving long-term opioid therapy (LTOT) for severe chronic pain from multiple conditions, including shoulder osteoarthritis following prior cervical spondylosis and diabetic neuropathy. She also has multiple sclerosis that has started to involve her diaphragm and lung volumes. She is prescribed long-acting morphine 30 mg three times a day, tramadol

Table 5 Words matter – person-first language	
Person-first language	**Stigmatizing and traumatizing language**
Person with substance use disorder	Addict, Drug abuser, Junkie, Drug seeker, Pill seeker
Person in recovery	Former addict
Drug misuse; Harmful use	Drug abuse
Substance use disorder	Drug habit
Being abstinent, being sober, not using, testing positive for substance use or consistent with abstinence	Being "clean" or "dirty" or "negative for substance use"
Heavy substance use over short time	Drug binge
Medications for Opioid Use Disorder	Opioid replacement therapy

Data from Olsen Y, Sharfstein JM. The opioid epidemic: what everyone needs to know: Oxford University Press, 20196; and Adults SAAO. Treatment Improvement Protocol (TIP) Series, No. 26. Center for Substance Abuse Treatment. Rockville (MD): Substance Abuse and Mental Health Services Administration (US) 1998.

100 mg every 6 hours as needed for pain, and lorazepam 0.5 mg daily as needed for anxiety. She has been asking for more pain medication as her pain is "not at all" controlled. Through virtual collaborative psychiatric care with a geriatric psychiatrist, Ms. T is diagnosed with mild OUD. Ms. T is educated about OUD and safely transitioned from morphine to buprenorphine 2 mg (along with naloxone) three times a day. Her tramadol and lorazepam are tapered off and duloxetine (for management of chronic pain) and cognitive behavior therapy for pain is initiated.

ROLE OF NALOXONE

PCPs should routinely prescribe naloxone to older adults with OUD to reduce the risk of opioid overdose death.[1] In addition, patients and/or caregivers may be able to obtain naloxone as permitted by the individual state through prescriptions, directly from a pharmacist, or as part of a community-based program. Naloxone is a strong affinity, full, competitive mu-opioid receptor antagonist and thus displaces opioid agonists, thereby reversing their effects.[21] Naloxone administration intranasally or parenterally (intramuscular, intravenous, subcutaneous) is the standard of care to reverse respiratory and central nervous system (CNS) depression that is known or suspected to be caused by an opioid overdose and thus prevent fatal overdose. Naloxone is lifesaving in these situations, and information has been issued by the Food and Drug Administration (FDA) to increase its use. It has a short half-life (2 hours) and thus, its effect although rapid and complete, is short-lasting (30–90 minutes).[21] Multiple doses of naloxone may be needed particularly when the overdose is caused by high potency opioids, like fentanyl.[21] A naloxone drip may be required to maintain safe respiration, especially if long-acting opioids (eg, methadone) have been used. Naloxone precipitates opioid withdrawal so that the person on waking up generally begins to experience distressing withdrawal symptoms.[21] PCPs should prescribe naloxone to patients with OUD and give prescriptions to their family, friends, and housemates after educating them about when and how to use it.[1] It is recommended that patients and people in close contact with them carry naloxone on their person for quick access if needed. After every situation that required naloxone administration in the community, emergency medical services should be activated to include emergency department care.[5]

OPIOID WITHDRAWAL MANAGEMENT

Opioid withdrawal produces extreme discomfort and hence medically managed opioid withdrawal is recommended.[7] This is generally done in an in-patient or residential setting but can also be safely done in an outpatient setting via telehealth. Symptoms include sweating, shaking, chills, body aches, yawning, large pupils, headache, craving, nausea, vomiting, abdominal cramping, diarrhea, insomnia, agitation, depression, anxiety, and other behavioral changes that can last for days to weeks[1] (see **Table 1**). Clinical opiate withdrawal scale may be used to monitor withdrawal symptoms.[22] Fear of withdrawal is a significant deterrent to stopping opioid use. Opioid withdrawal does not lead to delirium, so the presence of delirium suggests withdrawal of another substance (eg, benzodiazepines, alcohol).[6] In older adults, other causes of delirium (eg, infection) should also be looked for. The goal of withdrawal management in the context of OUD is to have a short period of withdrawal allowing for titration of buprenorphine or methadone that the patient can be stabilized and maintained on for relapse prevention.[6] If the patient chooses not to be on maintenance buprenorphine or methadone, then the goal of withdrawal management is to achieve a complete sustained withdrawal before adding naltrexone for relapse prevention.

Symptoms typically begin within 8 hours, peak at 48 to 72 hours, and resolve within 7 days.[23] Long-acting opioids (eg, methadone, fentanyl) may have delayed onset, delayed peak, and longer duration of withdrawal symptoms. A substantial proportion of individuals may have protracted withdrawal symptoms for additional 6 months.[20] Symptoms of menopause (eg, night sweats, achy joints) may be confused with that of opioid withdrawal.[24]

Nonopioid medications for symptomatic treatment include clonidine for treatment of sympathetic overactivity (eg, tachycardia, elevated blood pressure), loperamide for diarrhea, dicyclomine for abdominal cramps, nonsteroidal anti-inflammatory drugs (NSAIDs) for joint and muscle pain, and trazodone for insomnia. Muscle relaxants, antiemetics, and anxiolytics may also be used.[6] Lofexidine is approved by the FDA for the treatment of OUD and its mechanism of action is similar to clonidine. High cost of lofexidine is a barrier to its routine use. Successful opioid withdrawal by itself is not sufficient treatment and may paradoxically increase the risk of overdose, as well as a quick relapse if it is not followed by a comprehensive treatment of OUD that includes MOUD.[1]

Use of medications used to manage withdrawal carries an increased risk in older adults due to the prevalence of multiple serious multiple medical comorbidities.[7] PCPs can play a key role in collaboratively working with addiction treatment providers to ensure safe withdrawal management and minimize the risks of medications routinely used for the treatment of opioid withdrawal. For example, NSAIDs can also cause gastrointestinal bleeding, heart failure, and renal impairment in the elderly, and this needs to be carefully considered with their use.

MEDICATIONS FOR OPIOID USE DISORDER

Evidence shows that MOUDs (buprenorphine and methadone) are very effective in reducing opioid use and in reducing mortality even when used without psychosocial interventions and should not be withheld in patients who refuse or unable to obtain psychosocial interventions.[6,25] For some patients, medical management may suffice.[25] The FDA has approved three medications for the treatment of OUD: buprenorphine, methadone, and naltrexone.[26] These three medications together constitute MOUDs. Previously, the terms used were Medications for Addiction Treatment or Medication Assisted Therapy. Buprenorphine and methadone together constitute Opioid Agonist Therapy for OUD.

PCPs need to educate patients and family that methadone and buprenorphine do not produce a euphoric high in individuals with OUD due to the high tolerance to opioids that these individuals have developed and due to the unique pharmacodynamic and pharmacokinetic properties of these two opioids.[1] They instead minimize withdrawal symptoms and cravings, thereby promoting the normal functioning of the individual with OUD in relationships and activities of daily living. These medications are best seen as harm-reduction strategies. Most patients with OUD need MOUD for several years and some (eg, severe heroin addiction) for decades. The ultimate goal may be to wean the patient off these maintenance medications, but this decision needs to be made in collaboration with the patient, family, and team members.[7] Tapering of these medications needs to be done very slowly, over months or even years in some cases, only when there has been functional recovery, and when there are no ongoing significant psychosocial stressors or unstable comorbid conditions. Otherwise, the risk of relapse is considerable.[1]

In opioid-naïve patients, overdose-related deaths can occur with buprenorphine and methadone but is quite uncommon with buprenorphine use.[6] It mainly can happen with concurrent use of CNS depressants, primarily benzodiazepines. Overdose death with methadone is more of a concern which is greatly heightened by concurrent use of benzodiazepines and/or alcohol. Like other opioid medications, buprenorphine and methadone are sometimes diverted and misused.[1] Use of higher doses increases the risk of diversion.[5] Some diversion also occurs as patients try to manage withdrawal symptoms on their own. Diversion of methadone is more common with methadone prescribed for the treatment of pain than for the treatment of OUD. Buprenorphine and methadone control cravings better than naltrexone and hence are associated with better outcomes than naltrexone treatment, especially related to mortality reduction.[1,5] Patient's preference regarding the choice of MOUD needs to be considered.

BUPRENORPHINE

Buprenorphine is a high-affinity, partial mu-opioid agonist with slow dissociation, resulting in a lower risk of creating euphoria and lower risk of overdose death compared to full agonists.[1] It is approved by the FDA for the treatment of OUD. It is also used for opioid withdrawal management and pain management.[27] For OUD treatment and withdrawal management, it can be given once a day. For pain management, it may need to be given in three to four divided doses a day as its analgesic effect may wear off in 6 to 8 hours.[1]

Buprenorphine may be preferred over methadone and naltrexone for OUD treatment in older adults except in patients with injectable heroin-related OUD.[1] Buprenorphine has less risks than full opioid agonists (eg, oxycodone, morphine, fentanyl), but it is still a potent opioid with all the risks associated with opioid use listed in **Table 1**, and thus considered a high-risk medication in older adults.[7]

Unlike methadone, buprenorphine can be prescribed by PCPs in primary care and other office-based settings in the treatment of OUD, whereas methadone can only be used to treat OUD in federally qualified opioid treatment centers. Buprenorphine (being a partial agonist) can precipitate opioid withdrawal if receptors are bound by full agonists (heroin, prescription opioids) at the time of administration (Refer to case 2).[1] It should be started once opioid withdrawal symptoms develop in patients with OUD. Buprenorphine has a ceiling effect, and this can be a barrier to the treatment of individuals with higher opioid tolerance. In these individuals, initial transition to methadone and then to buprenorphine may be considered. It has higher affinity for mu-opioid receptors than other opioids and so impedes further opioid binding.[5] So, if a patient takes heroin or prescription opioids while on buprenorphine, they are unlikely to experience any euphoric effects. Buprenorphine does not require adjustment in individuals with renal failure. Compared with methadone, less is known about buprenorphine safety in older adults.[1] It is preferable to methadone because it is less likely to cause withdrawal symptoms, erectile dysfunction, constipation, and respiratory depression.[1,6]

For OUD treatment, the combination of buprenorphine and naloxone is preferred to buprenorphine alone to minimize the risk of diversion and intravenous self-administration and subsequent respiratory and CNS depression.[1] Older adults who have a significant decline in physical health or get transitioned to long-term care setting may be appropriate for taper and discontinuation of buprenorphine with continued close monitoring for relapse (eg, cravings are returning).[7]

Formulations and Dosing

Buprenorphine is available as buccal film, sublingual tablets, transdermal, long-acting injectable (weekly and monthly formulation) and 6-month buprenorphine subdermal implant.[6] Buprenorphine in combination with naloxone is available as buccal film (under the tongue or inside the cheek) and sublingual tablets. Naloxone has minimal bioavailability when taken buccally or sublingually, and hence it does not block the effect of buprenorphine unless taken parenterally.[5] Initial dosing begins with 2 mg in older adults (in combination with naloxone 0.5 mg) and, if well tolerated, the dose may be increased if withdrawal symptoms and/or cravings are not controlled. The final dose is generally lower in older adults than that needed for younger individuals. In younger individuals, the average dose range needed is around 16 to 24 mg once daily.

CASE 2: MS. S

Ms. S is a 61-year-old grandmother who relapsed on heroin after 5 years of recovery. Ms. S wants to babysit her granddaughter. Ms. S's daughter-in-law would not allow her to babysit until Ms. S was "clean." A friend of Ms. S offered her a buprenorphine film to help her get off heroin. Ms. S did not know much about buprenorphine and took it. After the first dose, she experienced severe heroin withdrawal symptoms. She called her PCP who informed her that buprenorphine could precipitate withdrawal and needed to be taken once withdrawal symptoms developed. PCP treated Ms. S's withdrawal symptoms and referred her to an outpatient opioid addiction treatment program in the community for comprehensive treatment along with MOUDs.

METHADONE

Methadone is a full mu agonist (1). It is approved by the FDA for treatment of OUD. It is also used to manage opioid withdrawal and for chronic, severe treatment refractory to pain.[27] For OUD treatment and withdrawal management, it can be given once a day. For pain management, it may need to be given in three to four divided doses a day (despite its long half-life) as its analgesic effect may wear off in 6 to 8 hours.[1] Patients receiving methadone for OUD cannot rely on once-a-day dosing for pain relief.

Methadone is a long-acting opioid. A dose on average lasts 24 to 36 hours (even longer in older adults).[1] Owing to its long half-life and its extremely variable and idiosyncratic dose response, it carries a higher risk of opioid overdose and overdose death compared with other opioids.[23] Owing to its NMDA receptor antagonistic activity, it may be used for opioid-induced hyperalgesia (OIH), as dysfunction in NMDA receptor activity has been implicated in the development of OIH.[6] Other opioids do not have NMDA antagonist property.[27] Methadone is relatively safe in individuals with renal failure compared with morphine for chronic severe treatment-refractory pain management. Methadone may be preferred over buprenorphine and naltrexone for older adults with severe OUD due to injectable opioid use[1] (Refer to Case 3).

The number of older adults in methadone treatment for OUD is growing.[20] Many older adults may be on methadone treatment for decades. Hence, although PCPs may not be prescribing methadone for OUD, they will need to learn the unique risks and benefits of methadone use in older adults.[7] Its use is associated with a significant reduction in opioid or illicit opioid cravings and does not cause euphoria in individuals with heroin addiction because it outcompetes heroin for opioid receptor binding.[1] This property also helps reduce heroin overdose and heroin overdose deaths because much of the effects of heroin are blocked by methadone.

Owing to the risk of drug–drug interactions, long half-life (and thus accumulation) and prolongation of QTc (and thus risk of arrhythmias), the use of methadone in older adults carries more risks than in younger adults and more risks compared with buprenorphine.[7,18] Pretreatment EKG and repeat EKG after 1 month of treatment with methadone are recommended. Owing to its long half-life, its idiosyncratic, variable, and unpredictable dose-response, and relatively shorter time taken to cause respiratory depression compared with pain relief, dangerous respiratory depression can occur if the dose is prematurely increased instead of waiting for 5 to 7 days or longer to reach a steady state. Because of the higher risk of sedation compared with buprenorphine, it should be avoided in older adults with severe respiratory or cardiac disease.[1,17]

Formulation and Dosing

Methadone is available as tablets and liquid. For OUD, it is given in the liquid form.[6] For pain, it is generally given in the tablet form, and the prescription should state that methadone is for pain.[1] For OUD, initial dosing in older adults should begin with 10 mg. The dose is slowly increased, and the final dose is generally lower than that needed for younger individuals. In younger individuals, doses of 100 mg of methadone or higher is not unusual.

CASE 3: MR. L

Mr. L is a 68-year-old nursing home resident, a retired veteran with chronic severe noncancer pain (due to multiple back surgeries, sciatica, arthritis). He also has a past history of heroin addiction, opioid overdose, and prescription misuse. Mr. L is on oxycodone 20 mg three times daily plus oxycodone 10 mg with acetaminophen 325 mg combination pill as needed every 6 hours for breakthrough pain. He has a long history of demanding more and more opioids for pain control. After his best friend recently passed away, he has been asking for all the as-needed medications almost every day. Through virtual collaborative psychiatric care with a geriatric psychiatrist, Mr. L is safely transitioned from oxycodone (both scheduled and as needed) to methadone 20 mg three times daily. Venlafaxine (for management of chronic pain) and grief counseling are initiated. The social worker helps Mr. L get connected to a local mutual aid support group and a peer support specialist.

NALTREXONE

Naltrexone is approved by the FDA for treatment of OUD, as well as alcohol use disorder (AUD).[6] For older adults with both OUD and AUD, naltrexone may be preferred over buprenorphine and methadone. Naltrexone is a full opioid antagonist. It is long acting and may be given every 2 to 3 days, especially in older adults although it is recommended as once-daily administration.[23] It should not be used in older adults requiring prescription opioids for pain relief. Naltrexone may precipitate significant opioid withdrawal symptoms in those taking opioids. To treat OUD, it is generally given at least 7 to 10 days after a medically supervised opioid withdrawal, and 10 to 14 days if withdrawing from buprenorphine or methadone.[1] This period is a high-risk period for relapse and thus, robust social support and use of psychological interventions are recommended to prevent relapse during this period.

Although high-quality studies of its use for OUD in older adults are lacking, naltrexone was found to be safe and effective for the treatment of AUD in older adults.[28] Nonadherence is more common with oral naltrexone than with buprenorphine or methadone and hence injectable once a month formulation is preferred. (Refer to Case 4).[5] Before giving long-acting injectable naltrexone, a trial of oral naltrexone should be considered to ensure that there is little risk for withdrawal symptoms or an allergic reaction. Naltrexone may cause liver dysfunction and hence PCPs should avoid naltrexone prescription in older adults with acute hepatitis or liver failure.[26]

Formulation and Dosing

Naltrexone is available as once-daily pill, as well as once a month injection (380 mg once a month), although the pill form is generally not recommended for the treatment of OUD mainly because of adherence issues compared with the injectable form. Typically, 25 mg naltrexone should be taken on day one and if it is tolerated well, from day two onwards 50 mg daily is recommended.

CASE 4: MR. A

Mr. A is a 66-year-old retired construction worker who has prescription OUD. His son wants him to get help but also tells him that he should not get on Suboxone (buprenorphine-naloxone combination pill) because that would be replacing one addictive drug with another addictive drug. Mr. A does not want methadone because he has seen a friend of his taking it and his friend has been partly nonadherent and in addition, at times his friend appears intoxicated. The PCP discusses the option of naltrexone and Mr. A agrees to a monthly injection of long-acting naltrexone.

BOLSTERING SOCIAL SUPPORT

Social support is critical to achieving and maintaining long-term recovery from OUD in older adults.[1] PCPs should diligently work to strengthen existing social networks and creating new networks. The latter includes recovery-oriented social networks (eg, mutual-aid support groups, peer recovery support specialists).[7] PCP should clarify the level of involvement of family and other support systems the patient would like to involve them throughout the treatment journey.

Mutual-aid support groups (eg, Narcotics Anonymous, Self-Management and Recovery Training, Celebrate Recovery) consist entirely of people who volunteer their time and typically have no official connection to addiction treatment centers.5 Such groups support abstinence and foster new social connections, a sense of belonging, and healthy lifestyles. Mutual-aid support groups may be critical to recovery for patients who cannot access treatment due to a lack of adequate health insurance coverage for addiction treatment.[25]

Older adults who take methadone may experience even more social isolation than older adults with other types of SUDs.[24] Older adults who have used opioids for many years may have severed ties with family and friends and lost friends who overdosed. People who take methadone may perceive significant stigma about their history of opioid use and their treatment from friends, family, and society.[1] Key reasons older adults with OUD may self-isolate are past experiences of being taken advantage of, fear of future loss, wish to avoid grief over the loss of family/friends, and past experiences of domestic violence.[7] It is recommended that PCPs have social workers in their practice who can address these concerns preemptively so that PCPs can then collaboratively work with their patients to build a nonopioid-using social network that supports MOUD as a pathway to recovery. Social workers can also help connect patients to peer-support specialists who can share their own experiences with addiction and recovery and also connect them to other resources; all of which have significant value.

ADDRESSING CO-OCCURRING DISORDERS

Identifying and treating all co-occurring disorders (not just optimal pain control) is essential if older adults with OUD are to achieve overall wellness.[7] PCPs can play a key role in optimally addressing co-occurring disorders. Older adults with OUD have a higher prevalence of depression, delirium, and dementia compared with older adults without OUD.[29] Older adults on methadone for OUD have higher rates of arthritis, hypertension, human immunodeficiency virus (HIV), and hepatitis C (HCV) compared to younger peers.[30,31] Opioids and naltrexone are metabolized by the liver and hence, their use in older adults with liver disease should be done with extreme caution and very low doses may need to be used. Caution is also needed in use of opioids in older adults with respiratory disorders (eg, chronic obstructive pulmonary disorder [COPD], obstructive sleep apnea [OSA], obesity hypoventilation syndrome, asthma).[7,17] Injection opioid use (eg, heroin) is the primary driver of the HIV and Hepatitis C epidemic. MOUDs can reduce HIV and HCV prevalence by reducing risk behaviors in people who inject heroin and other opioids. MOUDs also improve outcomes of HIV and HCV infection by promoting adherence to HIV and HCV treatment.[1]

LTOT is defined as the use of opioids on most days for more than 3 months.[32] There is no study that supports the use of LTOT for chronic noncancer pain.[27,32] There is one study that found LTOT for chronic moderate to severe hip, knee or back pain to be no better than nonopioid therapy and carried more risks than nonopioid therapy.[33] Hence, LTOT should be prescribed only in rare situations where the pain is severe, chronic, and treatment-refractory, and only if the benefits outweigh risks[1] based on the patient's medical and psychiatric comorbidity. Use of patient agreement forms are recommended before initiating LTOT.

Concurrent use of opioids and benzodiazepines and opioids and gabapentinoids (gabapentin, pregabalin) amongst 65 years and older is prevalent, generally prescribed by the same PCP, and poses a higher risk of overdose death, especially opioids and benzodiazepines.[1,27,34] Deprescribing of CNS depressants used concomitantly with opioids (eg, benzodiazepines, gabapentin, pregabalin, muscle relaxants, sedating antipsychotics [eg, quetiapine, olanzapine]) should be considered routinely.

Accidental overdose has been described in individuals taking both opioids and benzodiazepines, and this risk is even higher in individuals with certain medical comorbidities (eg, COPD, OSA).[7] Older adults also tend to misuse multiple medications (eg, opioids, benzodiazepines, hypnotics, muscle relaxants).[27,35] This in turn increases the risks of serious health consequences including death. PCPs should be diligent in avoiding the co-prescription of opioids and benzodiazepines and minimizing co-prescription of opioids and gabapentinoids.

SUMMARY

Managing OUDs in older adults takes a team due to multiple co-morbidities, polypharmacy, as well as limited supports. PCPs need to be vigilant in recognizing signs and symptoms, as well as taking preventative efforts. Ongoing advocacy is needed to support the reimbursement not only of medications but of supportive services. Expanded telehealth services need to be maintained in order to support older adults especially in medically underserved communities.

CLINICS CARE POINTS

- Primary care providers (PCPs) need to develop competency and confidence in prescribing as well as monitoring the use of buprenorphine and other treatment approaches for older adults with Opioid Use Disorder (OUD).

- Initiation of buprenorphine generally requires an interval of time without other opioids and development of some degree of opioid withdrawal symptoms, whereas initiation of naltrexone requires a much longer interval and opioids to be fully out of the system to avoid precipitated withdrawal.

- Concurrent use of opioids and benzodiazepines should be avoided because of the greatly increased risk of overdose and death, and prescribing opioids with any other medications or substances with central nervous system depressant properties (e.g., gabapentinoids, muscle relaxants, hypnotics, alcohol) also carries increased risk of overdose and death, and thus should be done with great caution or avoided.

- PCPs should educate patients and their family/friends/housemates regarding the use of naloxone and prescribe naloxone routinely for all patients who are prescribed opioids and for those who have OUD.

ACKNOWLEDGMENTS

The authors would like to express their deep gratitude to Dr Ingvild Olsen for her invaluable insights, edits, and guidance to improve our article.

DISCLOSURE

The authors have nothing to disclose.

REFERENCES

1. Olsen Y, Sharfstein JM. The opioid epidemic: what everyone needs to know. New York: Oxford University Press; 2019.
2. West NA, Severtson SG, Green JL, et al. Trends in abuse and misuse of prescription opioids among older adults. Drug and alcohol dependence 2015;149: 117–21.
3. Levi-Minzi MA, Surratt HL, Kurtz SP, et al. Under treatment of pain: a prescription for opioid misuse among the elderly? Pain Med 2013;14(11):1719–29.
4. Badrakalimuthu VR, Rumball D, Wagle A. Drug misuse in older people: old problems and new challenges. Adv Psychiatr Treat 2010;16(6):421–9.
5. Comer S, Cunningham C, Fishman MJ, et al. National practice guideline for the use of medications in the treatment of addiction involving opioid use. Am Soc Addict Med 2015;66:9–157.
6. Adults SAAO. Treatment improvement protocol (TIP) series, No. 26. center for substance abuse treatment. Rockville (MD): Substance Abuse and Mental Health Services Administration (US); 1998.
7. LaGrotta C. Treatment of opioid use disorder in the elderly. Curr Treat Options Psych 2020;7:531–43.
8. Larney S, Bohnert AS, Ganoczy D, et al. Mortality among older adults with opioid use disorders in the Veteran's Health Administration, 2000–2011. Drug Alcohol Depend 2015;147:32–7.
9. Wu L-T, Blazer DG. Illicit and nonmedical drug use among older adults: a review. J Aging Health 2011;23(3):481–504.
10. Webster LR, Webster RM. Predicting aberrant behaviors in opioid-treated patients: preliminary validation of the Opioid Risk Tool. Pain Med 2005;6(6):432–42.
11. Webster LR. Risk factors for opioid-use disorder and overdose. Anesth Analg 2017;125(5):1741–8.
12. Coambs RB, Jarry JL, Santhiapillai AC, et al. The SISAP: a new screening instrument for identifying potential opioid abusers in the management of chronic nonmalignant pain within general medical practice. Pain Res Manag 1996;1(3):155–62.
13. Belgrade MJ, Schamber CD, Lindgren BR. The DIRE score: predicting outcomes of opioid prescribing for chronic pain. J Pain 2006;7(9):671–81.

14. Butler SF, Budman SH, Fernandez KC, et al. Development and validation of the current opioid misuse measure. Pain 2007;130(1–2):144–56.

15. Butler SF, Fernandez K, Benoit C, et al. Validation of the revised Screener and Opioid Assessment for Patients with Pain (SOAPP-R). J Pain 2008;9(4):360–72.

16. de Vries F, Bruin M, Lobatto DJ, et al. Opioids and their endocrine effects: a systematic review and meta-analyses. J Clin Endocrinol Metab 2020;105(4):1020–9.

17. Rosen IM, Aurora RN, Kirsh DB, et al. Chronic opioid therapy and sleep: an American Academy of Sleep Medicine position statement. J Clin Sleep Med 2019; 15(11):1671–3.

18. Behzadi M, Joukar S, Beik A. Opioids and cardiac arrhythmia: a literature review. Med Princ Pract 2018;27(5):401–14.

19. Carew AM, Comiskey C. Treatment for opioid use and outcomes in older adults: a systematic literature review. Drug Alcohol Depend 2018;182:48–57.

20. Joshi P, Shah NK, Kirane HD. Medication-assisted treatment for opioid use disorder in older adults: an emerging role for the geriatric psychiatrist. Am J Geriatr Psychiatry 2019;27(4):455–7.

21. Ortega R, Nozari A, Baker W, et al. Intranasal naloxone administration. New Eng J Med 2021;384(12):e44.

22. Wesson DR, Ling W. The clinical opiate withdrawal scale (COWS). J Psychoactive Drugs 2003;35(2):253–9.

23. Sherman BJ, Hartwell KJ, McRae-Clark A, et al. Treatment of substance-related disorders. In: Schatzberg AF, Nemeroff CB, editors. The American Psychiatric Association publishing textbook of psychopharmacology. Arlington (VA): American Psychiatric Association Publishing; 2017. p. 1283–311.

24. Doukas N. Older adults prescribed methadone for opiate replacement therapy: a literature review. J Add Pre Med 2017;2(1):1–6.

25. Carroll KM, Weiss RD. The role of behavioral interventions in buprenorphine maintenance treatment: a review. Am J Psychiatry 2017;174:738–47.

26. Abuse S. Medications for opioid use disorder. Treatment improvement protocol (TIP) series 63. 2018

27. Gazelka HM, Leal JC, Lapid MI, et al. Opioids in older adults: indications, prescribing, complications, and alternative therapies for primary care. Mayo Clin Proc 2020;95(4):793–800.

28. Oslin D, Liberto JC, O'Brien J, et al. Tolerability of naltrexone in treating older, alcohol-dependent patients. The Am J Addict 1997;6(3):266–70.

29. Maree RD, Marcum ZA, Saghafi E, et al. A systematic review of opioid and benzodiazepine misuse in older adults. Am J Geriatr Psychiatry 2016;24(11):949–63.

30. Lofwall MR, Brooner RK, Bigelow GE, et al. Characteristics of older opioid maintenance patients. J Subst Abuse Treat 2005;28(3):265–72.

31. Rosen D, Smith ML, Reynolds CF III. The prevalence of mental and physical health disorders among older methadone patients. Am J Geriatr Psychiatry 2008;16(6):488–97.

32. Dowell D, Haegerich TM, Chou R. CDC guideline for prescribing opioids for chronic pain—United States, 2016. JAMA 2016;315(15):1–49.

33. Krebs EE, Gravely A, Nugent S, et al. Effect of opioid vs nonopioid medications on pain-related function in patients with chronic back pain or hip or knee osteoarthritis pain: the SPACE randomized clinical trial. JAMA 2018;319(9):872–82.

34. Musich S, Wang SS, Slindee LB, et al. Concurrent use of opioids with other central nervous system-active medications among older adults. Popul Health Manag 2020;23(4):286–96.

35. Tilly J, Skowronski S, Ruiz S. The opioid public health emergency and older adults. Greenville (NC): Administration for Community Living; 2017.

Illicit Drug Use in Older Adults: An Invisible Epidemic?

Ziad Ghantous, MD[a,b], Victoria Ahmad, MD[a,b], Rita Khoury, MD[a,b,c],*

KEYWORDS

- Illicit • Substance • Misuse • Elderly • Heroin • Cocaine • Stimulant
- Methamphetamine

KEY POINTS

- Analysis of longitudinal data from the National Surveys on Drug Use and Health (NSDUH) or other national databases has shown significant increases in the prevalence rates of heroin, cocaine, and stimulant use and misuse among those aged 50 years and older.
- Older users are vulnerable to specific triggering factors including physical symptoms such as pain, and psychiatric symptoms such as depression, anxiety, grief, loneliness, and social isolation.
- They are at increased risk for cardiovascular and cerebrovascular accidents, sexually transmitted infections, drug-drug interaction, cognitive impairment, and premature death while using heroin, cocaine, and other stimulants such as methamphetamines.
- Older users respond well to psychotherapy approaches, notably motivational interviewing, cognitive behavioral therapy, and contingency management. Although no pharmacotherapy is approved for the treatment of cocaine and other stimulant use disorders, there is solid evidence for use of opioid replacement therapy (methadone or buprenorphine) for heroin use disorder in older adults.
- There is a need to develop adapted screening tools for substance misuse in older adults and incorporate systematic assessment for these disorders in our routine practice. Treatment approaches need to be adapted to the physical, mental, and cognitive needs of older users, including telepsychiatry services and home visits when needed.

[a] University of Balamand, Faculty of Medicine, Youssef Sursock Street, PO Box 166378, Beirut, Lebanon; [b] Department of Psychiatry and Clinical Psychology, Saint Georges Hospital University Medical Center, Youssef Sursock Street, PO Box 166378, Beirut, Lebanon; [c] Department of Psychiatry and Behavioral Neuroscience, Saint Louis University School of Medicine, Missouri, USA
* Corresponding author. Department of Psychiatry and Clinical Psychology, Saint George Hospital University Medical Center, Youssef Sursock Street, PO Box 166378, Beirut, Lebanon.
E-mail address: rita.khoury@idraac.org

Clin Geriatr Med 38 (2022) 39–53
https://doi.org/10.1016/j.cger.2021.07.002
0749-0690/22/© 2021 Elsevier Inc. All rights reserved.

INTRODUCTION

Illicit drug use poses a worldwide public health problem. Since 1990, more countries are reporting increased injection drug use including heroin and cocaine, and increased manufacturing and trafficking of amphetamines and opium.[1]

The 2020 United Nations World Drug Report estimates 269 million people used illicit drugs at least once in the past year, among whom 57.8 million opioid users, 27 million amphetamine users, 20.5 million 3,4-methylenedioxy methamphetamine users, and 19 million cocaine users. Around 35.6 million people suffered from drug use disorders.[1]

With population aging, older adults currently constitute the fastest-growing segment of society in the United States and other developed countries.[2] Older adults encounter several challenges including loneliness, social isolation, grief, change in socioeconomic status, and exacerbation of their chronic medical problems, putting them at higher risk of developing substance use disorders among other psychiatric disorders.[3]

To date, the geriatric population has been marginalized within the field of substance use disorders, due to the relative rarity of the disorder compared with younger cohorts, and several misconceptions related to "old age" such as "maturing out" of addictions[4] or the unlikelihood to initiate illicit substance use after young adulthood.[5] However, current trends reveal that the geriatric share is increasing.[4,6,7] Thus, this population requires our attention as older users are unique in terms of risk factors, clinical characteristics, prognosis, and management approaches.

In this article, we will explore the geriatric trends in use and misuse of heroin, and stimulants including cocaine, amphetamines, and methamphetamines. We will review prevalence rates, comorbidities, and clinical considerations, in addition to assessment and management strategies relative to older adults.

There is no formal definition for "older drug user." Although the official retirement age ranges between 60 and 65 years, lower cut-offs ranging between 40 and 50 years have been used in the literature. This is because illicit drug users suffer from serious medical complications as they grow older, and have a higher risk of mortality, at least two decades earlier than nonusers. To enlarge the scope of our review, we included studies that used an age cut-off of 40 years and older to define an older drug user.[8]

EPIDEMIOLOGY

In a nationally representative sample comprising 10,953 community-dwelling American adults aged 50 years and older, past-year prevalence rates of substance use disorders were calculated based on data extracted from the public files of the 2005 to 2006 National Surveys on Drug Use and Health (NSDUH). This survey is based on self-reports from noninstitutionalized Americans during in-person interviews, using the DSM-IV criteria.[9] The past-year prevalence rate for heroin use disorder was 0.05% (SD = 0.03), compared with 0.18% (SD = 0.05) for cocaine use disorder and 0.01% (SD = 0.01) for stimulant use disorder. The number of older adults having illicit drug use disorder was too small in this sample to be able to generate reliable prevalence rates.[9]

Heroin

Most studies have found that approximately 30% of heroin users continue to use heroin into old age, reiterating that heroin use disorder is a chronic relapsing/remitting condition.[10] To further study the longitudinal trend of heroin use in the United States, data were collected from the Treatment Episode Data Set for Admissions (TEDS-A) between 2004 and 2015 involving 400,421 adults aged 55 years and older. The proportion of older adults with primary heroin use more than doubled between 2012 and 2015 (P<.001); these individuals were increasingly men (P<.001), African American (P<.001), and used via the intranasal route (P<.001), suggesting a possible switch from prescription opioids to cheaper heroin to meet their increasing need for opioids.[11]

Gender differences were studied in a qualitative study grouping 38 older American heroin users (aged 50 years and older): women significantly expressed more than men guilt and remorse while describing the toll of the drug use on their children. However, losing loved ones because of drugs was a common central theme in the narratives of both men and women, triggering relapse, increased use, or sometimes recovery from heroin use.[10] Heroin users can be divided based on age of initiation into those who started using in young adulthood (before age 30 years) versus those who began later in life (after age 30 years).[7,12] When compared with early-onset users, late-onset users were more likely white, female, middle class, highly educated, married or divorced/widowed, and living independently. They were also more frequently heroin users, but less likely to inject.[7,12]

According to Wall and colleagues (2018), drug use is an age-graded behavior, depending on which substance is more readily available at the time of a generation's highest risk of initiation, that is, their early adulthoods. The use of heroin peaked in the early 1970s compared with other substances.[5] This coincided with the current geriatric population's early years; reports show that this cohort (people born between the late 1940s and early 1960s) has the highest prevalence of injection drug use ever reported in the United States.[13] According to Cicero and colleagues (2014), more than 80% of those who initiated opioid misuse in the 1960s started with heroin.[14] In addition, the current prescription opioid epidemic must be taken into consideration, with several estimates indicating that there will be more "late-onset" heroin users consisting of those who transition from prescription pills or initiate heroin later in life. In fact, Lynch and colleagues (2021) pointed to an increase of about 60% in all first admissions for people aged 55 years and older over a 10-year period, with heroin being the second (after alcohol) most cited primarily abused drug for all admissions to substance abuse treatment among patients more than 50 years.[7,15,16] Several papers corroborated the increasing rate of heroin use and overdoses[14,17–19] in recent years, specifically among 55 to 64 and ≥65 years.[6] Multiple factors are incriminated: First, the older cohort is more likely to have chronic pain diagnoses, disabilities, multiple comorbidities, and thus, opioid prescriptions.[19,20] The interrelatedness of prescription pills and heroin has been studied, pointing to a gateway drug effect with people transitioning to the latter for various reasons including the greater availability and affordability of heroin,[5,14,21–23] urbanicity,[24] ease of use, and the euphoric reward of heroin compared to pills.[14] Second, loneliness in older adults is associated with increased illicit substance use.[25–27] Anderson and Levy (2003) shed light on the phenomenon of marginalization of older heroin users. As they age, and in conformity with social norms, their position in the illicit drug culture varies, as they continue to participate, largely unseen. This phenomenon exacerbates their loneliness and depression.[28]

Cocaine

Longitudinal trends for cocaine use and misuse were studied by comparing 2 sets of data derived from the National Epidemiologic Survey on Alcohol and Related Conditions (NESARC) between 2001 to 2002 and 2012 to 2013. Although rates of cocaine use and cocaine use disorder remain lower among older than younger individuals in

2001 to 2002 and 2012 to 2013, significant increases in cocaine use and misuse were only seen among the group of older individuals: the 12-month prevalence of cocaine use and use disorder among those aged 45 years and older increased from 0.14% to 0.49% and 0.07% to 0.19%, respectively. Therefore, there is a need to follow the baby-boomer cohort closely to anticipate continuous increase in the prevalence of cocaine use disorder among the geriatric population.[29] Prevalence rates of cocaine use were found to be even higher when research studies used objective assessment measures such as urine drug screens: in the emergency department setting of an academic suburban community hospital, 2.3% of American adults aged 65 years and older were found to screen positive for cocaine. These findings highlight stigma and shame related to reporting illicit drug use (cocaine here) among seniors. In addition, a chart review of 117 American veterans aged 50 years and older treated for cocaine misuse revealed that 14.5% used cocaine for the first time after the age of 50 years.[30]

Other Stimulants (Methamphetamines/Amphetamines)

Based on data from the 2015 to 2018 NSDUH, the prevalence rate for past-year methamphetamine use was found to be 3.2/1000 (95% confidence interval [CI], 2.8–3.9) among those aged 50 years and older.[31] Previous NSDUH reports in the early 2000s showed that methamphetamine users were mostly aged 18 to 25 years, whereas analysis of more recent data shows that a large proportion of methamphetamine users are in the 35-year-old age group and older, suggesting a cohort effect, and the importance of following the trend for use as this population ages.[32]

Methamphetamine use was found to be particularly increased among older adults in trauma clinic settings: in a retrospective cohort study involving 5278 patients aged 55 years and older, 8% were methamphetamine users as reflected by their positive urine drug screen in 2018, compared with 2% in 2009.[33]

According to data from the NSDUH, lifetime nonmedical prescription stimulant use was found to increase from 5.2% (4.46–5.94) to 7.2% (6.27–8.01) between 2002 to 2003 and 2012 to 2013 among adults aged 50 years and older. Past-year nonmedical prescription stimulant use increased from 0.1% (0.04–0.23) to 0.3% (0.14–0.45) between the 2 dates.[34] These numbers remained stable in the following years as shown by analysis of 2015 to 2016 NSDUH data among Americans aged 50 years and older: prescription stimulant misuse without use disorder was 0.3% (95% CI, 0.19–0.35) and prescription stimulant use disorder was 0.1% (95% CI, 0.04–0.12).[35] Adults aged 55 years and older constituted 10.6% (95% CI, 9.2–11.9) of those presenting to an emergency department for any amphetamine-type stimulant overdose, across the United States in 2017.[36]

PHYSICAL AND PSYCHIATRIC COMORBIDITIES
Heroin

Physical diseases found in older heroin users include hypertension (between 50% and 58% of cases), obesity in 54%, dyslipidemia in 22%, diabetes in 7% to 18%, cardiovascular disease between 18% and 53%, gastrointestinal diseases between 21% and 27%, cirrhosis between 7% and 14%, chronic lung disease in 22%, and arthritis in 29% to 54%. Comorbid-reported sexually transmitted diseases include hepatitis C in 24% to 94% of cases, hepatitis B in 85.6%, human immunodeficiency virus (HIV) in up to one-third of cases, and syphilis in 3.8% of cases.[16,37,38] Similarly, data from the United Kingdom show a steady increase in both the prevalence and incidence rates of hepatitis C among current and ex-drug injectors, as they grow older. The impact of this phenomenon is under-recognized, given that deaths related to these infections are not classified under United Kingdom or European definitions as drug-related deaths and are therefore not counted in official figures.[39]

Screening for psychiatric disorders was performed in a sample of 140 older adults (age 50–70 years) who attended methadone clinics (64.3% men; 52.1% African American) using the DSM-III criteria. The past-year prevalence of having any mental health disorder in this population was 57%. The 3 most common disorders were major depression, generalized anxiety disorder, and post-traumatic stress disorder (32.9%, 29.7%, and 27.8%, respectively). In addition, 57.7% of the respondents reported having fair to poor physical health, assessed using the Composite International Diagnostic Interview, the SF-12 health survey version.[38]

Another cross-sectional study conducted in a methadone maintenance clinic in New York showed that older attendees (aged 55 years and older) had poor quality of life, similar to younger attendees, as reflected by the Overall Social Support scale, the Personal Well-Being Index, and the Satisfaction with Life Scale. Surprisingly, despite an increase in their medical and psychiatric problems, they had increasingly limited contact with a primary care physician, as they were growing older.[40]

It is believed that cumulative heavy opioid use is associated with a slightly significant increase in dementia risk (hazards ratio of 1.29 [CI, 1.02–1.62]). Anatomopathological research has shown that opioids may be associated with brain neuropathologic findings similar to what is seen in Alzheimer's disease on autopsy.[41] This effect may be mediated by modulation of microglia and neuroinflammation caused by opioids. No data are available regarding the direct effect of heroin on the brain and cognitive decline as heroin users get older. Heroin, like other opioids,[42] is associated with delirium in older adults, which is by itself a risk factor for developing dementia.

Stimulants

Cocaine and other stimulants are associated with vasoconstriction, and increased cardiovascular risk, notably hypertension, myocardial infarction, arrhythmias, cerebral infarcts, and intracerebral hemorrhage.[43,44] These effects will complicate preexisting cardiovascular and neurologic disorders in this population, putting the patients at increased risk of premature death. Furthermore, attention and working and visual memory can be severely impaired in cocaine users, leading to exacerbation of dementia in older users.[45] In a recent study, cocaine misuse was associated with accelerated aging: the annual rate of global gray matter volume loss in cocaine-dependent individuals was found to be almost twice the rate of healthy volunteers (3 mL/y [SD 0.49] vs 1.69 mL [SD 0.41], respectively). This difference was found to be statistically significant, even after excluding subjects with comorbid alcohol use disorder ($P = .013$).[46] Cocaine is also associated with disruption of sleep pattern and architecture, which warrants special consideration in older adults.[40] Like heroin injections, crack cocaine administered intravenously is associated with increased risk of infection and sexually transmitted diseases via syringe sharing.[47]

Methamphetamine is rapidly taken by various organs such as the lungs, brain, liver, pancreas, stomach, and kidneys, explaining a wide range of complications such as pulmonary hypertension and kidney failure.[48]

In a sample of 5278 adults aged 55 years and older who were admitted to a trauma center, methamphetamine users were significantly more likely to require surgical intervention (35% vs 17% in nonusers), mechanical ventilation (15% vs 7% in nonusers), and a longer hospitalization (6.5 vs 3.6 days in nonusers).[33]

There is a link between methamphetamine use and engaging in risky sexual behavior and therefore increasing the risk of contracting HIV. In a study involving 482 Australian homosexual men aged 40 years and older, of whom 13% reported methamphetamine use, HIV-positive men were 2.5 times more likely to report methamphetamine use than HIV-negative men.[49]

Studies in animals and humans have shown a detrimental effect of methamphetamine on the central nervous system, leading to cortical volume loss through inflammatory changes and microglial activation.[50] Methamphetamine was shown to specifically damage dopaminergic neurons in the striatum and substantia nigra, increasing the likelihood of developing Parkinson's disease.[51] The combined effect of prior methamphetamine use and HIV seropositivity was found to be detrimental on several domains of neurocognitive functioning in adults aged 50 years and older.[52]

In addition, methamphetamine use has been associated with emergence of psychosis (hallucinations, paranoid delusions, and disorganized behavior) that can further exacerbate cognitive decline.[53]

SCREENING/DIAGNOSTIC TOOLS

The DSM-5 criteria for substance use disorder constitute the gold-standard diagnostic assessment tool. Two or more criteria met within a 12-month period are required to establish the diagnosis: hazardous use, social/interpersonal problems related to use, neglected major roles to use, withdrawal, tolerance, used larger amounts/longer duration, repeated attempts to quit/control use, much time spent using, physical/psychological problems related to use, activities given up to use, and craving.[54] These criteria need to be adapted in older adults for several reasons: first, cognitive impairment impacts adequate self-reporting of the amounts consumed as well as craving sensations. It also impacts their judgment and capacity to realize the extent of the disorder and hazardous situations where they have been consuming. Role obligations that drug users fail to fulfill may not exist for older adults in the same way as for younger adults because of life-stage transitions, such as retirement. The role obligations more common in late life are caregiving for an ill spouse or family member, such as a grandchild. Tolerance and withdrawal symptoms may develop at very low doses, given the sensitivity of the receptors to drug use.[55]

Although there are various screening tools for substance use disorders in the general population, there is a dearth of tools that have been validated for the geriatric population.[4,16] The CAGE-AID shown in **Box 1** is a brief (4-questions) and practical screening tool for alcohol and substance use. However, it fails to distinguish between current and lifetime use, which is specifically problematic when screening older patients who may have a history of substance misuse, but not necessarily a current problematic one.[56] The Alcohol, Smoking, and Substance Involvement Screening Test (ASSIST) developed by the World Health Organization is another brief, 8-question questionnaire that screens for tobacco, alcohol, cannabis, cocaine, amphetamine-type stimulants (including

---

Box 1
CAGE-AID, a brief screening tool for substance use disorders

CAGE-AID
1. Have you ever felt that you should cut down on your drug use?
2. Have people annoyed you by criticizing your drug use
3. Have you ever felt bad or guilty about your drug use?
4. Have you ever used drugs first thing in the morning to steady your nerves or to get rid of a hangover (eye opener)?

Data from Brown RL, Rounds LA. Conjoint screening questionnaires for alcohol and other drug abuse: criterion validity in a primary care practice. *Wis Med J.* 1995;94(3):135-140

Table 1	
The alcohol, smoking and substance involvement screening test (ASSIST)	
	ASSIST
Q1	Asks about which substances have ever been used in the client's lifetime
Q2	Asks about the frequency of substance use in the past 3 mo, which gives an indication of the substances that are most relevant to current health status
Q3	Asks about the frequency of experiencing a strong desire or urge to use each substance in the last 3 mo
Q4	Asks about the frequency of health, social, legal, or financial problems related to substance use in the last 3 mo
Q5	Asks about the frequency with which use of each substance has interfered with role responsibilities in the past 3 mo
Q6	Asks if anyone else has ever expressed concern about the client's use of each substance and how recently that occurred
Q7	Asks whether the client has ever tried to cut down or stop use of a substance, and failed in that attempt, and how recently that occurred
Q8	Asks whether the client has ever injected any substance and how recently that occurred

Data from Humeniuk RE, Henry-Edwards S, Ali RL, Poznyak V, Monteiro M. The Alcohol, Smoking and Substance Involvement Screening Test (ASSIST) Manual for Use in Primary Care. World Health Organization; 2010; and Who.int. Accessed May 31, 2021. https://apps.who.int/iris/bitstream/handle/10665/44320/9789241599382_eng.pdf?sequence=1.

ecstasy), inhalants, sedatives, hallucinogens, opioids, and "other drugs" (shown in **Table 1**). A risk score is provided for each substance, and scores are grouped into "low risk," "moderate risk," or "high risk." The risk score determines the level of intervention recommended (brief intervention or brief intervention plus referral to specialist treatment).[57] It takes 5 to 10 minutes to administer and is recommended for use in primary care settings. Khan and colleagues (2012) have validated a French version of ASSIST in the elderly.[58] One hundred patients were recruited, ages ranging between 65 and 93 with a mean of 77.8 ± 7.5 years (72% women). The ASSIST was compared to the Addiction Severity Index (ASI), the Alcohol Use Disorders Identification Test (AUDIT), and the Revised Fagerstrom Tolerance Questionnaire-Smoking. The ASSIST alcohol scores showed large positive correlation with the ASI and AUDIT scores ($r = 0.73$ and $P<.0005$, $r = 0.8$ and $P<.0005$, respectively), while the ASSIST tobacco scores also showed large positive correlation with the Fagerstrom questionnaire ($r = 0.8$ and $P<.0005$). However, correlation was not possible for ASSIST and ASI opioid scores because of the lack of enough data. The ASSIST questionnaire showed good internal consistency for the total substance involvement substance score (Cronbach's α coefficient of 0.72 [95% CI 2 {0.63, 0.79}, $P<.0005$]), as did the ASSIST scores for alcohol, tobacco, and sedatives (0.66, 0.74, and 0.89, respectively). Sensitivity and specificity estimates could not be performed because of lack of sufficient data.[59] This tool was also effectively used in a sample of 210 Australian participants aged 60 years and older (mean age 81.9 years, 63.3% women) without dementia or delirium to detect illicit substance use in the past 3 months.[58]

CHALLENGING ASSESSMENT

Substance use disorders are underdiagnosed in older adults because of several factors including ageism (stigma, prejudice, and stereotypes against older people), denial, isolation, and shame of older adults, in addition to the lack of training of health care workers, and the complex atypical presentations that are often disguised as other geriatric syndromes.[60,61] For example, perimenopausal symptoms, such as hot flashes, outbreaks of sweat and fatigue are often identical to opioid withdrawal symptoms leading to misidentification of the latter.[62] Assessment of older adults requires a meticulous, supportive, and nonconfrontational interviewing style, with specific, detailed questions about use and frequency in the context of overall health and behavior. Physicians practicing in the primary care and emergency settings need to routinely screen for these disorders in their daily practice. **Box 2** shows a thorough assessment evaluation of older adults with respect to substance use disorders. A thorough investigation into risk factors, medical and psychiatric comorbidities, as well as drug-drug interactions is needed.

MANAGEMENT

Older adults are often barred from treatment because of misconceptions related to ageism. Studies have shown that older adults have the capacity to change and respond well to motivational interviewing and can successfully demonstrate physical and psychological long-term recovery.[61]

A comprehensive and holistic approach is needed to engage and provide care to this population with complex physical, cognitive, and social limitations.

Heroin

Current guidelines for heroin use disorder recommend opioid maintenance treatments (OMT) such as buprenorphine and methadone.[60]

Methadone is a full mu-opioid receptor agonist, the first to be approved in replacement or maintenance therapy, and linked to decreased cue-induced craving, improved mood, regained connections to loved ones,[16] and reduced risk of death.[63,64] On the contrary, buprenorphine is a high affinity partial mu-opioid receptor agonist that was found to reduce risk of death and decrease symptoms of dysphoria in those with opioid use disorder.[63,64] Given its partial agonist activity, buprenorphine is

---

Box 2
Assessment of older adults with substance use disorder

Identify precipitating factors: grief, isolation, retirement, immobility, mental disorders, medical problems, pain, sleep disturbances, and trauma

Inquire about somatic symptoms: tremor, dizziness, falls, incontinence, memory problems, and pain

Obtain collateral history from family/caregivers/family doctor/hospital discharge summaries

Screen for comorbid psychiatric disorders including depression, anxiety, suicidality, and post-traumatic stress disorder

Conduct a systematic cognitive assessment to rule out neurocognitive disorders, and determine mental capacity

Screen for comorbid medical conditions including renal and liver impairment, and sexually transmitted infections

Check for drug-drug interaction

Data from Rao R, Crome I, Crome P, Iliffe S. Substance misuse in later life: challenges for primary care: a review of policy and evidence. Prim Health Care Res Dev. 2019;20(e117):e117; Dürsteler-MacFarland KM, Vogel M, Wiesbeck GA, Petitjean SA. There is no age limit for methadone: a retrospective cohort study. Subst Abuse Treat Prev Policy. 2011;6(1):9.

associated with a ceiling effect causing less respiratory depression and has lower overdose potential compared with methadone.[65]

In a study of older adults in Singapore, methadone maintenance treatment was shown to be cost-effective in treating elderly opium users (mean age 74.8 years). No other illicit drugs were detected in the participants' urine samples, 3 years into the treatment. Although the typical dose of methadone for the treatment of heroin misuse ranges between 60 and 120 mg, only a mean dose of 9 mg was used in this older group, for safety reasons. Psychiatrists collaborated closely with caregivers/family members, providing monthly prescriptions of methadone, to be administered by caregivers.[66]

Studies in older adults in methadone maintenance treatment have shown that around 30% of patients suffer from major depressive disorder, leading to impairment in their functioning and on treatment adherence.[67] Management of psychiatric comorbidities including depression, anxiety, and post-traumatic stress disorder in the geriatric population is mandatory to improve functional status and retention in treatment. In addition, it is important to incorporate a protocol for suicide ideation assessment among older adults with depression, in methadone maintenance treatment (aged 50+ years).[68] Low-dose buprenorphine (0.2–16 mg/d) has been studied for treatment-resistant depression in adults aged 50 years and older in a pilot randomized controlled trial, showing significant improvement of depression as measured by the Montgomery Asberg Depression Rating Scale (MADRS) at 8 weeks.[69] This drug might thus be beneficial as OMT and adjunctive antidepressant treatment in certain patients.

Management of chronic pain in older adults is necessary. Strategies include scheduled acetaminophen, antidepressants such as selective serotonin and noradrenaline reuptake inhibitors (SNRI) or tricyclics. Duloxetine (SNRI) is Food and Drug Administration approved for neuropathic pain, fibromyalgia, and musculoskeletal pain.[70] Newer antiepileptics such as gabapentin and pregabalin can be particularly useful for neuropathic pain.[71] Furthermore, nonpharmacological approaches such as physical therapy, pain rehabilitation, and mind-body therapies have a significant role in the management of chronic pain in older adults.[72]

In terms of tolerability and safety of OMT, there is no evidence of age-related alterations in methadone metabolism. However, dose adjustments may be required for patients taking other medications known to interact with methadone (eg, antiviral medications, antidepressants, antiepileptics, etc.) or for patients with severe liver or kidney disease.[73] Owing to cumulative effects, caution is needed when respiratory-depressant medications such as benzodiazepines are co-prescribed with either methadone or buprenorphine.[62] Potential complications associated with methadone use include prolongation of the corrected QT interval, high drug-drug interactions via the cytochrome P450 (CYP)-3A4 enzyme, and a long elimination half-life, especially in older adults producing greater toxicity. Buprenorphine is, in theory, a better option for older adults: it does not cause prolonged QTc, nor requires dose adjustment in renal failure.[72] It may also be a safer option than methadone for individuals with severe cardiac or respiratory illnesses. Although methadone clinics have federal regulations and require regular counseling sessions, toxicology screens and same-day screening requests, buprenorphine can be managed in outpatient settings, which may be more practical for older adults.[74]

Other adverse events related to opioids are gastrointestinal, mainly nausea and constipation. Although opioids are known to worsen cognition, OMT in patients who are not opioid naïve had a neutral effect on cognition.[75]

Despite studies showing the effectiveness of OMT in treating opioid use disorder in older adults,[16,76] there are several barriers hindering access to maintenance treatments in this population such as the long-held preference for abstinence models over OMT programs,[63,77,78] the misconception of maturing out of addiction with age,[4] in addition to increased isolation and loss of personal relationships leading to decreased initiation and retention in OMT programs.[16,79,80]

Stimulants

There is no approved pharmacologic treatment for cocaine or stimulant use disorders. The latest meta-analysis that reviewed the efficacy of antidepressants, antiepileptics such as topiramate, dopamine agonists, and antipsychotics did not find any statistically significant superiority over placebo. There may be a promising role of slow-acting psychostimulant therapy, but more robust studies are needed to ascertain this finding.[81] The standard of care treatment is psychosocial: it involves individual and group therapy. The strongest evidence exists for contingency management, which is a behavioral intervention that uses a voucher-based reinforcement, also known as voucher-based reinforcement therapy (VBRT). In this type of therapy, on achieving a set therapy goal such as obtaining a negative urine drug screen, patients receive vouchers that can be exchanged for goods, services housing, employment, and so forth.[82] This can especially be useful in older adults who are socially isolated and have limited family and financial support. A combination of VBRT and cognitive behavioral therapy can help sustain a significant period of abstinence and prevent relapse. Unfortunately, there are limited treatment programs specifically designed for older adults.[56,83]

SUMMARY

Illicit substance use disorders are under-reported, underdiagnosed, and undertreated in older adults.

Older users have complex and unique clinical presentations and needs. Given the higher prevalence of physical and mental health comorbidities compared with younger substance users, a holistic and multidisciplinary approach is needed to improve outcomes and quality of life. Barriers to identify these disorders should be attenuated such as stigma, prejudice, ageism, and lack of training of health care workers.[80] A systematic screen for substance use/misuse in aging baby boomers should be performed by all health care workers working with older adults including primary care physicians, geriatricians, psychiatrists (geriatric/addiction specialists), pain specialists, and psychotherapists. More research is needed to determine true prevalence figures, and adapt age-sensitive screening tools, in addition to facilitate access to treatment modalities through specialized clinics, telepsychiatry services, and home visits.

CLINICS CARE POINTS

- Older illicit drug users are at increased risk for cardiovascular and cerebrovascular accidents, premature death, sexually transmitted infections, drug-drug interaction, cognitive impairment, depression and psychosis while using heroin, cocaine, and other stimulants such as methamphetamines
- Older users respond well to psychotherapy approaches, notably motivational interviewing, cognitive behavioral therapy, and contingency management. While no pharmacotherapy is approved for treatment of cocaine and other stimulant use disorders, there is solid evidence for use of opioid replacement therapy (methadone or buprenorphine) for heroin use disorder in older adults.

- There is a need to adapt specific screening tools for substance misuse in older adults and incorporate systematic assessment for these disorders in routine geriatric and psychiatric practice.
- Treatment approaches need to be adapted to the physical, mental and cognitive needs of older users, including telepsychiatry services and home visits when needed.

DISCLOSURE

The authors have nothing to disclose.

REFERENCES

1. Degenhardt L, Hall W. Extent of illicit drug use and dependence, and their contribution to the global burden of disease. Lancet 2012;379(9810):55–70.
2. US Census Bureau. A snapshot of the fast-growing U.S. older population. Available at: https://www.census.gov/library/stories/2018/10/snapshot-fast-growing-us-older-population.html. Accessed May 30, 2021.
3. Arndt S, Schultz SK. Epidemiology and demography of alcohol and the older person. In: Flint A, Merali Z, Veccarino F, editors. Substance use and older people. Ottawa (Canada): John Wiley & Sons, Ltd; 2014. p. 75–90.
4. Simoni-Wastila L, Yang HK. Psychoactive drug abuse in older adults. Am J Geriatr Pharmacother 2006;4(4):380–94.
5. Wall M, Cheslack-Postava K, Hu M-C, et al. Nonmedical prescription opioids and pathways of drug involvement in the US: generational differences. Drug Alcohol Depend 2018;182:103–11.
6. Scholl L, Seth P, Kariisa M, et al. Drug and opioid-involved overdose deaths - United States, 2013-2017. MMWR Morb Mortal Wkly Rep 2018;67(5152): 1419–27.
7. Lynch A, Arndt S, Acion L. Late- and typical-onset heroin use among older adults seeking treatment for opioid use disorder. Am J Geriatr Psychiatry 2021;29(5): 417–25.
8. Gaulen Z, Alpers SE, Carlsen S-EL, et al. Health and social issues among older patients in opioid maintenance treatment in Norway. Nordisk Alkohol Nark 2017; 34(1):80–90.
9. Blazer DG, Wu L-T. The epidemiology of substance use and disorders among middle aged and elderly community adults: national survey on drug use and health. Am J Geriatr Psychiatry 2009;17(3):237–45.
10. Hamilton AB, Grella CE. Gender differences among older heroin users. J Women Aging 2009;21(2):111–24.
11. Huhn AS, Strain EC, Tompkins DA, et al. A hidden aspect of the U.S. opioid crisis: rise in first-time treatment admissions for older adults with opioid use disorder. Drug Alcohol Depend 2018;193:142–7.
12. Boeri MW, Sterk CE, Elifson KW. Reconceptualizing early and late onset: a life course analysis of older heroin users. Gerontologist 2008;48(5):637–45.
13. Armstrong GL. Injection drug users in the United States, 1979-2002: an aging population: an aging population. Arch Intern Med 2007;167(2):166–73.
14. Cicero TJ, Ellis MS, Surratt HL, et al. The changing face of heroin use in the United States: a retrospective analysis of the past 50 years: a retrospective analysis of the past 50 years. JAMA Psychiatry 2014;71(7):821–6.

15. Lofwall MR, Schuster A, Strain EC. Changing profile of abused substances by older persons entering treatment. J Nerv Ment Dis 2008;196(12):898–905.

16. Rosen D, Hunsaker A, Albert SM, et al. Characteristics and consequences of heroin use among older adults in the United States: a review of the literature, treatment implications, and recommendations for further research. Addict Behav 2011;36(4):279–85.

17. Rudd RA, Paulozzi LJ, Bauer MJ, et al. Increases in heroin overdose deaths - 28 States, 2010 to 2012. MMWR Morb Mortal Wkly Rep 2014;63(39):849–54.

18. Hedegaard H, Chen L-H, Warner M. Drug-poisoning deaths involving heroin: United States, 2000-2013. NCHS Data Brief 2015;190:1–8.

19. Lagisetty P, Zhang K, Haffajee RL, et al. Opioid prescribing history prior to heroin overdose among commercially insured adults. Drug Alcohol Depend 2020; 212(108061):108061.

20. Weiss AJ, Heslin KC, Barrett ML, et al. Opioid-related inpatient stays and emergency department visits among patients aged 65 years and older, 2010 and 2015. In: HCUP statistical brief #244. 2018. Available at: https://www.hcup-us.ahrq.gov/reports/statbriefs/sb244-Opioid-Inpatient-Stays-ED-Visits-Older-Adults.pdf.

21. Jones CM, Logan J, Gladden RM, et al. Vital signs: demographic and substance use trends among heroin users - United States, 2002-2013. MMWR Morb Mortal Wkly Rep 2015;64(26):719–25.

22. Compton WM, Jones CM, Baldwin GT. Relationship between nonmedical prescription-opioid use and heroin use. N Engl J Med 2016;374(2):154–63.

23. Papp J, Vallabhaneni M, Morales A, et al. Take -home naloxone rescue kits following heroin overdose in the emergency department to prevent opioid overdose related repeat emergency department visits, hospitalization and death- a pilot study. BMC Health Serv Res 2019;19(1):957.

24. Pear VA, Ponicki WR, Gaidus A, et al. Urban-rural variation in the socioeconomic determinants of opioid overdose. Drug Alcohol Depend 2019;195:66–73.

25. Boehlen F, Herzog W, Quinzler R, et al. Loneliness in the elderly is associated with the use of psychotropic drugs: loneliness and psychotropic drugs in the elderly. Int J Geriatr Psychiatry 2015;30(9):957–64.

26. Taipale HT, Bell JS, Uusi-Kokko M, et al. Sedative load among community-dwelling people aged 75 years and older: a population-based study: a population-based study. Drugs Aging 2011;28(11):913–25.

27. Polenick CA, Cotton BP, Bryson WC, et al. Loneliness and illicit opioid use among methadone maintenance treatment patients. Subst Use Misuse 2019;54(13): 2089–98.

28. Anderson TL, Levy JA. Marginality among older injectors in today's illicit drug culture: assessing the impact of ageing: marginality among older injectors. Addiction 2003;98(6):761–70.

29. Kerridge BT, Chou SP, Pickering RP, et al. Changes in the prevalence and correlates of cocaine use and cocaine use disorder in the United States, 2001-2002 and 2012-2013. Addict Behav 2019;90:250–7.

30. Chait R, Fahmy S, Caceres J. Cocaine abuse in older adults: an underscreened cohort: letters to the editor. J Am Geriatr Soc 2010;58(2):391–2.

31. Jones CM, Compton WM, Mustaquim D. Patterns and characteristics of methamphetamine use among adults — United States, 2015–2018. MMWR Morb Mortal Wkly Rep 2020;69(12):317–23.

32. Chen L-Y, Strain EC, Alexandre PK, et al. Correlates of nonmedical use of stimulants and methamphetamine use in a national sample. Addict Behav 2014;39(5): 829–36.

33. Benham DA, Rooney AS, Calvo RY, et al. The rising tide of methamphetamine use in elderly trauma patients. Am J Surg 2021. https://doi.org/10.1016/j.amjsurg. 2021.02.030.

34. Schepis TS, McCabe SE. Trends in older adult nonmedical prescription drug use prevalence: results from the 2002–2003 and 2012–2013 National Survey on Drug Use and Health. Addict Behav 2016;60:219–22.

35. Compton WM, Han B, Blanco C, et al. Prevalence and correlates of prescription stimulant use, misuse, use disorders, and motivations for misuse among adults in the United States. Am J Psychiatry 2018;175(8):741–55.

36. Vivolo-Kantor AM, Hoots BE, Seth P, et al. Recent trends and associated factors of amphetamine-type stimulant overdoses in emergency departments. Drug Alcohol Depend 2020;216(108323):108323.

37. Hser Y-I, Gelberg L, Hoffman V, et al. Health conditions among aging narcotics addicts: medical examination results. J Behav Med 2004;27(6):607–22.

38. Rosen D, Smith ML, Reynolds CF III. The prevalence of mental and physical health disorders among older methadone patients. Am J Geriatr Psychiatry 2008;16(6):488–97.

39. Beynon CM, Roe B, Duffy P, et al. Self reported health status, and health service contact, of illicit drug users aged 50 and over: a qualitative interview study in Merseyside, United Kingdom. BMC Geriatr 2009;9(1):45.

40. Rajaratnam R, Sivesind D, Todman M, et al. The aging methadone maintenance patient: treatment adjustment, long-term success, and quality of life. J Opioid Manag 2018;5(1):27.

41. Dublin S, Walker RL, Gray SL, et al. Prescription opioids and risk of dementia or cognitive decline: a prospective cohort study. J Am Geriatr Soc 2015;63(8): 1519–26.

42. Swart LM, van der Zanden V, Spies PE, et al. The comparative risk of delirium with different opioids: a systematic review. Drugs Aging 2017;34(6):437–43.

43. Yarnell SC. Cocaine abuse in later life: a case series and review of the literature. Prim Care Companion CNS Disord 2015;17(2). https://doi.org/10.4088/PCC. 14r01727.

44. Rivers E, Shirazi E, Aurora T, et al. Cocaine use in elder patients presenting to an inner-city emergency department. Acad Emerg Med 2004;11(8):874–7.

45. Dokkedal-Silva V, Kim LJ, Galduróz J, et al. Cocaine use by older populations, sleep quality, and associated risks. Rev Bras Psiquiatr 2018;40(4):459.

46. Ersche KD, Jones PS, Williams GB, et al. Cocaine dependence: a fast-track for brain ageing? Mol Psychiatry 2013;18(2):134–5.

47. Carvalho HB de, Seibel SD. Crack cocaine use and its relationship with violence and HIV. Clinics (Sao Paulo) 2009;64(9):857–66.

48. Volkow ND, Fowler JS, Wang G-J, et al. Distribution and pharmacokinetics of methamphetamine in the human body: clinical implications. PLoS One 2010; 5(12):e15269.

49. Lyons A, Pitts M, Grierson J. Methamphetamine use in a nationwide online sample of older Australian HIV-positive and HIV-negative gay men: methamphetamine use and older gay men. Drug Alcohol Rev 2013;32(6):603–10.

50. Thanos PK, Kim R, Delis F, et al. Chronic methamphetamine effects on brain structure and function in rats. PLoS One 2016;11(6):e0155457.

51. Granado N, Ares-Santos S, Moratalla R. Methamphetamine and Parkinson's disease. Parkinsons Dis 2013;2013:308052.

52. Iudicello JE, Morgan EE, Gongvatana A, et al. Detrimental impact of remote methamphetamine dependence on neurocognitive and everyday functioning in older

but not younger HIV+ adults: evidence for a legacy effect? J Neurovirol 2014; 20(1):85–98.

53. Searby A, Maude P, McGrath I. Growing old with ice: a review of the potential consequences of methamphetamine abuse in Australian older adults. J Addict Nurs 2015;26(2):93–8.

54. Hasin DS, O'Brien CP, Auriacombe M, et al. DSM-5 criteria for substance use disorders: recommendations and rationale. Am J Psychiatry 2013;170(8):834–51.

55. Han BH, Moore AA. Prevention and screening of unhealthy substance use by older adults. Clin Geriatr Med 2018;34(1):117–29.

56. Kuerbis A, Sacco P, Blazer DG, et al. Substance abuse among older adults. Clin Geriatr Med 2014;30(3):629–54.

57. Humeniuk R, Ali R, Babor TF, et al. Validation of the alcohol, smoking and substance involvement screening test (ASSIST). Addiction 2008;103(6):1039–47.

58. Khan R, Chatton A, Thorens G, et al. Validation of the French version of the alcohol, smoking and substance involvement screening test (ASSIST) in the elderly. Subst Abuse Treat Prev Policy 2012;7(1):14.

59. Draper B, Ridley N, Johnco C, et al. Screening for alcohol and substance use for older people in geriatric hospital and community health settings. Int Psychogeriatr 2015;27(1):157–66.

60. Le Roux C, Tang Y, Drexler K. Alcohol and opioid use disorder in older adults: neglected and treatable illnesses. Curr Psychiatry Rep 2016;18(9):87.

61. Rao R, Crome I, Crome P, et al. Substance misuse in later life: challenges for primary care: a review of policy and evidence. Prim Health Care Res Dev 2019; 20(e117):e117.

62. Dürsteler-MacFarland KM, Vogel M, Wiesbeck GA, et al. There is no age limit for methadone: a retrospective cohort study. Subst Abuse Treat Prev Policy 2011; 6(1):9.

63. Salmond S, Allread V. A population health approach to America's opioid epidemic. Orthop Nurs 2019;38(2):95–108.

64. Kakko J, Alho H, Baldacchino A, et al. Craving in opioid use disorder: from neurobiology to clinical practice. Front Psychiatry 2019;10:592.

65. Whelan PJ, Remski K. Buprenorphine vs methadone treatment: a review of evidence in both developed and developing worlds. J Neurosci Rural Pract 2012; 3(1):45–50.

66. Guo S, Winslow M, Manning V, et al. Monthly take-home methadone maintenance regime for elderly opium-dependent users in Singapore. Ann Acad Med Singapore 2010;39(6):429–34.

67. Rosen D, Engel R, McCall J, et al. Using problem-solving therapy to reduce depressive symptom severity among older adult methadone clients: a randomized clinical trial. Res Soc Work Pract 2018;28(7):802–9.

68. McCall J, Brusoski M, Rosen D. Research with older adult methadone clients: the importance of monitoring suicide ideation. J Gerontol Soc Work 2017;60(6–7): 458–70.

69. Karp JF, Butters MA, Begley AE, et al. Safety, tolerability, and clinical effect of low-dose buprenorphine for treatment-resistant depression in midlife and older adults. J Clin Psychiatry 2014;75(8):e785–93.

70. Skljarevski V, Zhang S, Iyengar S, et al. Efficacy of duloxetine in patients with chronic pain conditions. Curr Drug Ther 2011;6(4):296–303.

71. Viniol A, Ploner T, Hickstein L, et al. Prescribing practice of pregabalin/gabapentin in pain therapy: an evaluation of German claim data. BMJ Open 2019;9(3): e021535.

72. Gazelka HM, Leal JC, Lapid MI, et al. Opioids in older adults: indications, prescribing, complications, and alternative therapies for primary care. Mayo Clin Proc 2020;95(4):793–800.

73. Volpe DA, Xu Y, Sahajwalla CG, et al. Methadone metabolism and drug-drug interactions: in vitro and in vivo literature review. J Pharm Sci 2018;107(12):2983–91.

74. Joshi P, Shah NK, Kirane HD. Medication-assisted treatment for opioid use disorder in older adults: an emerging role for the geriatric psychiatrist. Am J Geriatr Psychiatry 2019;27(4):455–7.

75. Dagtekin O, Gerbershagen HJ, Wagner W, et al. Assessing cognitive and psychomotor performance under long-term treatment with transdermal buprenorphine in chronic noncancer pain patients. Anesth Analg 2007;105(5):1442–8.

76. Crome I, Sidhu H, Crome P. No longer only a young man's disease–illicit drugs and older people. J Nutr Health Aging 2009;13(2):141–3.

77. Larochelle MR, Bernson D, Land T, et al. Medication for opioid use disorder after nonfatal opioid overdose and association with mortality: a cohort study. Ann Intern Med 2018. https://doi.org/10.7326/m17-3107.

78. Volkow ND, Frieden TR, Hyde PS, et al. Medication-assisted therapies–tackling the opioid-overdose epidemic. N Engl J Med 2014;370(22):2063–6.

79. Conner KO, Rosen D. "you're nothing but a junkie": multiple experiences of stigma in an aging methadone maintenance population. J Soc Work Pract Addict 2008;8(2):244–64.

80. Smith ML, Rosen D. Mistrust and self-isolation: barriers to social support for older adult methadone clients. J Gerontol Soc Work 2009;52(7):653–67.

81. Ronsley C, Nolan S, Knight R, et al. Treatment of stimulant use disorder: a systematic review of reviews. PLoS One 2020;15(6):e0234809.

82. Kampman KM. The treatment of cocaine use disorder. Sci Adv 2019;5(10):eaax1532.

83. National Survey of Substance Abuse Treatment Services (N-SSATS). Data on Substance Abuse treatment facilities. Samhsa.gov. 2019. Available at: https://www.samhsa.gov/data/report/national-survey-substance-abuse-treatment-services-n-ssats-2019-data-substance-abuse. Accessed May 30, 2021.

Hallucinogen Use and Misuse in Older Adults

Wm Maurice Redden, MD*, Saif-Ur-Rahman Paracha, MD,
Quratulanne Sheheryar, MD

KEYWORDS

- Hallucinogen • Psychedelic • LSD • PCP • Ketamine • Older adults

INTRODUCTION

Hallucinogens, also known as psychedelics ("mind manifesting"), are substances that have been used for over a millennium.[1] These drugs produce sensory distortions and have been used by various cultures for several reasons ranging from religious ceremonies to recreational activities. The term hallucinogen is used to describe compounds, such as psilocybin and D-lysergic acid diethylamide (LSD), based on the belief that these drugs elicit hallucinations. It has been argued that, at the doses commonly taken recreationally, rarely will one experience frank hallucinations.[2]

The US federal law placed strict control of these substances in 1970. This greatly halted research efforts on the benefits of these drugs. Subsequently, there are limited comparable data available on hallucinogenic drug abuse in older adults. The evidence suggests that although illegal drug use is relatively rare among older adults compared with younger adults and adolescents, there is a growing problem of misuse and abuse of prescription drugs with abuse potential. At present, these data do not include hallucinogen use.

Recent studies have renewed interest in hallucinogens and their potential therapeutic use.[3–6] Most of the studies do not include a significant number of patients that would be classified as elderly (aged 65 years and greater). Most publications discussing or classifying hallucinogen use refer to older adults aged 50 or greater.

WHAT ARE HALLUCINOGENS?

Psychedelic plants, such as mescaline and psilocybin, have been used for religious, healing, and celebratory purposes for more than six thousand years.[7,8]

Hallucinogens, as a drug category, include an enormous range of pharmacologic substances, with mechanisms of action ranging from N-methyl-D-aspartate (NMDA) antagonism (ie, phencyclidine [PCP]), muscarinic receptor antagonism (ie, scopolamine), k opioid agonism (ie, salvinorin A), mixed action monoamine release (ie,

Division of Geriatric Psychiatry, Department of Psychiatry & Behavioral Neuroscience, St. Louis University School of Medicine, 1438 South Grand Boulevard, St Louis, MO 63104, USA
* Corresponding author.
E-mail address: maurice.redden@health.slu.edu

Clin Geriatr Med 38 (2022) 55–66
https://doi.org/10.1016/j.cger.2021.07.007
geriatric.theclinics.com
0749-0690/22/© 2021 Elsevier Inc. All rights reserved.

3,4-methylenedioxymethamphetamine [MDMA]), and a common main agonistic action on 5-HT2A receptors (ie, LSD).[9]

On a fundamental level, hallucinogens can be described as substances that predominantly cause changes in thought, perception, and mood with minimal intellectual or memory impairment.[10] They are typically divided into 2 types: classical and dissociative drugs (**Table 1**).

The classical hallucinogens comprise 3 main chemical classes: the plant-derived tryptamines (eg, psilocybin), phenethylamines (eg, mescaline), and the semisynthetic ergolines (eg, LSD).[11]

Psilocybin (4-phosphoryloxy-*N,N*-dimethyltryptamine) comes from certain types of mushrooms found in tropical and subtropical regions of South America, Mexico, and the United States. Mescaline (Peyote) is a small, spineless cactus used to make synthetic LSD. It was first synthesized in 1938 by a Swiss natural products chemist, Dr Albert Hofmann,[12] who was looking for possible therapeutic uses of ergot derivatives.

In addition, there are synthetic ergolines, which include MDMA (also known as ecstasy), as well as 251-NBOMe, which has similarities to both LSD and MDMA but is much more potent. Also, of note, the drug ecstasy is often classified a hallucinogen because of its ability to cause subjective effects to distort time and induce distortions in visual perceptions as well as enhance enjoyment from tactile experiences. However, it also has some structural and psychoactive properties of stimulants.

N,N-Dimethyltryptamine (DMT) is a powerful chemical found naturally in some Amazonian plants. Ayahuasca is a tea made from such plants.[13] It is a brew used in traditional spiritual ceremonies by indigenous people of the Amazon Basin and has been legalized for ritual purposes in Brazil since 1987. It is often prepared with mixture of 2 plants, one containing the psychoactive substance DMT, a serotonin and sigma-1 receptor agonist, and another containing reversible monoamine oxidase inhibitors.[14]

The dissociative drugs include the following:

PCP was developed in the 1950s as a general anesthetic for surgery, but it is no longer used for this purpose because of serious side effects. PCP has various slang names, such as Angel Dust, Hog, Love Boat, and Peace Pill.[13]

Ketamine is a noncompetitive NMDA-receptor antagonist and a dissociative anesthetic developed in 1962. Much of the ketamine sold on the streets is stolen from veterinary offices. It is primarily sold as a powder or as pills, but it is also available as an injectable liquid. Ketamine is snorted or sometimes added to drinks as a date-rape drug. Slang names for ketamine include Special K and Cat Valium.[13]

Salvia (*Salvia divinorum*) is a plant common to southern Mexico, Central America, and South America. Salvia is typically ingested by chewing fresh leaves or by drinking

Table 1 Hallucinogens[9–13]	
Classical	**Dissociative**
• Psilocybin known as magic mushrooms • Mescline (Peyote) • ᴅ-Lysergic acid diethylamide (LSD) • Methylenedioxymethamphetamine (MDMA): known as ecstasy • 251-NBOMe is a synthetic hallucinogen with similarities to both LSD and MDMA • *N,N*-dimethyltryptamine (DMT) • Ayahuasca tea	• Phencyclidine (PCP) • Ketamine: anesthetic • Dextromethorphan cough suppressant

their extracted juices. The dried leaves of salvia can also be smoked or vaporized and inhaled. Popular names for salvia are Diviner's Sage, Maria Pastora, Sally-D, and Magic Mint.[13]

Epidemiology

The Controlled Substances Act of 1970 was a federal act passed by the US Congress that placed comprehensive drug control policy under federal control. This included the laws related to the manufacturing, possession, sale, import, and distribution of certain substances. The initial bill passed by Congress included a list of substances, but the Drug Enforcement Agency and the Food and Drug Administration (FDA) have regulated the ongoing restrictions in partnership.[15]

They classified hallucinogens as schedule 1 drugs, which are defined as having no accepted medical use and potential to cause significant harm and dependence. Even during inception, this ruling was viewed as being unscientific. Despite the lack of scientific evidence to support the initial claims, these drugs have remained schedule 1 drugs as originally ruled.

Therefore, by the late 1960s and early 1970s, the scientific inquiries fell out of favor because classical psychedelics were being used outside of medical research and in association with the emerging recreational use.

The lifetime prevalence rates and 12-month prevalence rates for total drug use disorders for age group 45 to 64 are 9.7% and 2.5%, respectively. For those aged 65 and up, lifetime and past-year prevalence rates reach 2% and 0.8%, respectively.[16]

In 2010, an estimated 32 million people reported a lifetime use of LSD, psilocybin, mescaline, or peyote. The prevalence of psychedelic use was low among people aged 65 and older, being reported as 1.3%.[17] In a follow-up study, it was shown that the lifetime hallucinogen use is prevalent and highly comorbid with other substance use and psychiatric disorders. In a study published in 2019 (data were collected from April 2012 through June 2013), the 12-month prevalence and lifetime hallucinogen use were 0.62% and 9.32%, respectively, for all ages. For the age group 45 to 64 years, lifetime prevalence was 11.32%, with a 12-month prevalence of 0.08%. In those aged 65 years and older, rates were 1.74% for lifetime and 0% for the past-year use.[18]

The overall LSD use in the United States increased to 56.4% from 2015 to 2018. For those aged 50 years or older, there was an increase from 1.83% to 2.66%. There was a significant increase (223.1%) in LSD use in older adults (particularly those aged 35–49) and a 45% increase in individuals greater than 50 years of age.[19]

MECHANISMS OF ACTION

It has been hypothesized that the hallucinogenic effects of these drugs in humans are mediated in whole or in part via 5-HT2 receptors.[20] It is the agonistic action on 5-HT2A receptors that produces the psychedelic effect, independently of dopamine stimulation.[21]

Both PCP and ketamine exert their effects by antagonism of NMDA receptors. This may also play a role in their potential therapeutic benefits.[22]

EFFECTS ON MIND AND BODY

The effects of hallucinogens are heavily dependent on the expectations of the user ("set") and the environment ("setting") in which the use takes place. Indeed, no clinician experienced with these substances would fail to consider set and setting as primary determinants of the experience. Thus, expectations and environments that would foster religious or spiritual experiences increase the probability of the drug producing such an effect. Conversely, use in a nonstructured, unwise, or recreational way can have unpredictable and even disastrous psychological consequences.[23]

Results suggest that even in today's context of "recreational" drug use, psychedelics, such as LSD and psilocybin, when taken at higher doses, continue to induce mystical experiences in many users.[24]

There was a study in which low doses of LSD were given to older healthy volunteers to measure the safety risks. A total of 48 subjects were divided into 1 of 4 dose groups: 5 μg, 10 μg, or 20 μg LSD, or placebo. They received their assigned study dose on 6 separate occasions over 21 days within a 96-hour interval. Overall, results suggest that administration of low-dose LSD carried no safety risk and was well tolerated during the limited 21-day period studied. Evaluation of cognitive and behavioral outcomes indicates a favorable safety profile overall, further supporting the feasibility of periodic LSD administration up to 20 μg.[25]

Healthy patients (with the oldest being aged 51) were given 200 μg of LSD, and they experienced pronounced alteration in waking consciousness, including visual perceptual alterations, audiovisual synesthesia, and positively experienced derealization and depersonalization. LSD did not induce pronounced anxiety and overall produced high ratings of good drug effects and low ratings of bad drug effects.[26]

ACUTE EFFECTS

Clinical effects of hallucinogens range from somatic symptoms, such as dizziness, to major psychological symptoms, including visual hallucinations[27] (**Table 2**).

Although hallucinogens are relatively safe physiologically and are not considered drugs of dependence, their use involves unique psychological risks. The most likely risk is overwhelming distress during drug action ("bad trip"), which could lead to potentially dangerous behavior.[28]

Of note, the *Diagnostic and Statistical Manual of Mental Disorders* (Fifth Edition) makes distinction between PCP use disorders and other hallucinogen use disorders. There is also a notable difference with intoxication symptoms because of PCP versus other hallucinogens (shown in **Table 3**). One main difference is that the other hallucinogens, such as LSD, exert their physical effects via stimulation of the sympathetic nervous system. This can lead to dilated pupils, tachycardia, increased cardiovascular risk, insomnia, and increased blood pressure.[29]

These adverse effects may be amplified in older patients, who may also have multiple medical comorbidities. For example, dizziness may put them at increased risk of falls, or increased blood pressure may increase their risk of stroke or cardiovascular events.

Table 2 Effects from hallucinogens[27–29]	
Mind and Body	**Short- and Long-Term Effects**
• Mystical experience • Ego dissolution • Positively experienced derealization and depersonalization • Dizziness and weakness	• Blurred vision and paresthesia • Difficulty focusing but improving hearing • Mood swings • Visual hallucinations • Flashback/hallucinogen persisting perception disorder (HPPD)

Table 3 Intoxication[50]	
Phencyclidine (PCP)	**Other Hallucinogens**
• Behavioral changes, such as belligerence, aggressivity, and agitation • Nystagmus • Hypertension or tachycardia • Numbness • Ataxia • Dysarthria • Muscle rigidity • Seizures or coma • Hyperacusis	• Behavioral changes, such as anxiety, depression, "losing one's mind," or paranoia • Depersonalization or derealization • Hallucinations or illusions • Pupillary dilation • Tachycardia • Sweating and palpitations • Blurring vision • Tremor • Incoordination

POTENTIAL BENEFITS

Over the past several years, a phenomenon known as "microdosing" has become popular, leading to several observational studies demonstrating benefits and challenges related to the use of these substances.[30]

"Microdosing" is associated with enhanced mood and work performance, via increased energy, concentration, and creativity. Also, most individuals who engage in microdosing had at some point in their life used psychedelics as the regular recreational dose.[31] This could lead one to hypothesize that older people who engaged in recreational use of hallucinogens when younger might engage in using microdoses of hallucinogens to help improve mood and cognition in late life.

More recently, several human studies have been conducted that are driving further research into the possible therapeutic benefits of hallucinogens in the management of psychiatric disorders. Some of these are mentioned in later discussion.

Depression

Hallucinogens have been a subject of curiosity in the treatment of depression for many decades. Psilocybin has been of particular interest in this regard in recent years. Therapeutically, psilocybin has made subjects more vividly aware of memories and promotes an overall feeling of well-being as well as reverses negative cognitive biases or distortions. Therefore, in clinical trials, psilocybin is often used to target anxiety-related disorders and depression.[32] Acutely, treatment with psilocybin has been shown to decrease amygdala reactivity during emotion processing and that this was associated with an increase of positive mood in healthy volunteers. These findings may be relevant to the normalization of amygdala hyperactivity and negative mood states in patients with major depression.[33] Larger double-blind, randomized, placebo-controlled, crossover trials have shown acute and sustained decrease in anxiety and depression symptoms after therapeutic administration of psilocybin in patients with cancer.[34]

Although LSD was an area of interest in the mid-twentieth century, statistically significant efficacy in the treatment of depression was not found. A recent study examined the effects of low-dose LSD versus placebo via functional MRI scans. Remarkably, the findings revealed extensive changes in brain connectivity and a subjective change in mood positivity.[35]

Other smaller studies have revealed a reduction in impulsive behavior, psychological distress, and suicidal ideation in patients with hallucinogen use. In comparison, other illicit drug use has been associated with an increase in such behavior.[36]

NMDA receptor-modulating drugs, such as ketamine, have been used in the treatment of depression. Safety and tolerability profiles with ketamine at low single dose are generally good in depressed patients. However, there is a lack of data concerning ketamine with repeated administration at higher doses.[6]

In a recent double-blind, controlled, multiple-crossover study, ascending doses of ketamine were given to older adults with treatment-resistant depression. There were a total of 16 participants 60 years or older. They were given single dose of 0.1, 0.2, 0.3, 0.4, or 0.5 mg/kg in separate treatment sessions at least a week apart. A single dose of midazolam 0.01 mg/kg was used as an active control treatment and was randomly inserted within the first 3 treatment sessions. Seven of 14 randomized controlled trial (RCT)-phase completers remitted with ketamine treatment. In addition, 2 of the 7, who did not remit after a single treatment (in the RCT phase), did attain remission after multiple treatments in the open-label phase. The investigators suggest that some who do not remit after 1 treatment may yet attain a meaningful remission after repeated treatments given at the same dose level at this treatment frequency. Ketamine was well tolerated, with the most common side effects being transient dizziness, fatigue, and blurred vision.[37]

In a small study, intravenous ketamine was given to older adults with treatment-resistant depression to evaluate its safety and efficacy. Six patients, aged 65 to 82, were given subanesthetic ketamine at a dose of 0.5 mg/kg delivered intravenously over 40 minutes. Five patients showed a robust response, after the acute phase, but they all lost the response over time. However, none returned to their baseline level of depression.[38]

The clinical use of ketamine has been increasing. Intranasal (S)-ketamine has recently been approved for depression by the FDA. It could be a promising treatment in depressed patients with suicidal ideation.[39]

Thus far, there have been limited results with the use of esketamine in older patients. In a double-blind randomized study, patients aged 65 and older with treatment-resistant depression were given either esketamine nasal spray combined with oral antidepressant (esketamine/antidepressant) or oral antidepressant and placebo nasal spray (antidepressant/placebo). There was no statistically significant change in the Montgomery-Åsberg Depression Rating Scale from baseline to day 28, as the primary endpoint. Further studies are thus needed to better evaluate the efficacy of esketamine in the elderly.[40]

In addition, there is some evidence supporting the safety and therapeutic value of single-dose ayahuasca, to help treat depression.[41]

Anxiety and Posttraumatic Stress Disorders

As mentioned above, psilocybin has been shown to also reduce symptoms of anxiety in patients with cancer.[41] A small modified double-blind study revealed a marked decrease in symptoms of obsessive-compulsive disorder in 9 patients when treated with psilocybin in a controlled environment.[42] MDMA has also shown promise in the treatment of anxiety disorders when used with adjunctive psychotherapy. MDMA-assisted psychotherapy with close follow-up, monitoring, and support has been shown to be effective in the treatment of chronic, treatment-resistant posttraumatic stress disorder.[43]

Substance Use Disorders

Psilocybin has been shown to be effective and safe in the treatment of alcohol dependence. It helped to decrease cravings and increase in length of abstinence from alcohol use.[44] Positive results were also seen when psilocybin was used for smoking cessation.[45]

Treatment with LSD has been studied and has shown benefit in the management of alcohol use disorder. A meta-analysis of RCT to evaluate the clinical efficacy of LSD in the treatment of alcohol use disorder revealed that a single dose of LSD, in conjunction with various alcoholism treatment programs, is associated with a decrease in alcohol misuse.[5]

Neurocognitive Disorders

Some preliminary findings indicate that psychedelic drugs have effects on several cognitive/affective processes that are altered in older adulthood. These findings also propose that hallucinogen use increases neuroplasticity, neurogenesis, connectedness, and mystical experiences, which have been reasoned to underlie cognitive/affective changes.[46] In addition, functional MRI studies have shown increased connectivity between regions with high 5HT2A receptor density following LSD administration, suggesting that reorganizing of dysfunctional neural circuitry is an important component of the neuroplastic effects of 5HT2A receptor agonists.[47] Furthermore, hallucinogens have been shown to have strong anti-inflammatory properties, which may represent an opportunity in the prevention of Alzheimer disease, which has largely been thought to result from inflammatory processes.[48]

Recently, a study has been proposed to evaluate the effects of repeated low doses of psilocybin and LSD on cognitive and emotional dysfunctions in Parkinson disease.[49]

DIAGNOSTIC CRITERIA FOR PHENCYCLIDINE AND OTHER HALLUCINOGEN USE DISORDER

Its main features include a problematic pattern of use that leads to clinically significant impairment or distress.[50] One can have tolerance without having dependence (**Box 1**).

LONG-TERM EFFECTS

It was initially thought that the lifetime use of psychedelics would not cause any undesirable long-term effects. However, new evidence shows that use within the past year may lead to negative mental health outcomes, including serious psychological distress, mental health treatment (inpatient, outpatient, medication, felt a need but did not receive), or symptoms of major mental health disorder.[51] However, in a review from contemporary studies (1994 to present), long-term effects were associated with use of classical hallucinogens. These effects include sustained changes in personality/attitudes, depression, spirituality, affect/mood, anxiety, well-being, substance use, meditative practices, and mindfulness.[52]

Evidence supports the association of LSD use with panic reactions, prolonged schizoaffective psychoses, and posthallucinogen perceptual disorder, the latter being present continuously for up to 5 years.[53] MDMA use has been associated with depression, anxiety, elevated impulsiveness, and memory deficits. The symptoms may persist for up to 2 years after cessation.[54]

The terms flashback and hallucinogen persisting perception disorder (HPPD) are often used interchangeably in professional literature. This unique condition is described as the recurrence of some of the symptoms that appeared during the intoxication after the immediate effect of the hallucinogen has worn off. This recurring syndrome, mainly visual, has not been clearly understood, appreciated, or distinguished from other clinical entities by clinicians. Flashback is usually a short-term,

---

Box 1
Diagnostic criteria for phencyclidine and other hallucinogen use disorder[50]

A problematic pattern of phencyclidine (or other hallucinogen) use leading to clinically significant impairment or distress, as manifested by at least 2 of the following, occurring within a 12-month period:

1. Phencyclidine (or other hallucinogen) is often taken in larger amounts or over a longer period than was intended.

2. There is a persistent desire or unsuccessful efforts to cut down or control phencyclidine (or other hallucinogen) use.

3. A great deal of time is spent in activities necessary to obtain phencyclidine (or other hallucinogen), use phencyclidine, or recover from its effects.

4. Craving, or a strong desire or urge to use phencyclidine (or other hallucinogen).

5. Recurrent phencyclidine (or other hallucinogen) use resulting in a failure to fulfill major role obligations at work, school, or home (eg, repeated absences from work or poor performance related to phencyclidine use; phencyclidine-related absences, suspensions, or expulsions from school; or neglect of children or household).

6. Continued phencyclidine (or other hallucinogen) use despite having persistent or recurrent social or interpersonal problems caused or exacerbated by the effects of phencyclidine (eg, arguments with a spouse about consequences of intoxication or physical fights).

7. Important social, occupational, or recreational activities are given up or reduced because of phencyclidine (or other hallucinogen) use.

8. Recurrent phencyclidine (or other hallucinogen) use in situations in which it is physically hazardous (eg, driving an automobile or operating a machine when impaired by a phencyclidine).

9. Phencyclidine (or other hallucinogen) use is continued despite knowledge of having a persistent or recurrent physical or psychological problem that is likely to have been caused or exacerbated by phencyclidine.

10. Tolerance, as defined by either of the following:
    a. A need for markedly increased amounts of phencyclidine to achieve intoxication or desired effect.
    b. A markedly diminished effect with continued use of the same amount of phencyclidine.

Withdrawal symptoms and signs are not established for phencyclidines and other hallucinogens, so this criterion does not apply.

---

nondistressing, spontaneous, recurrent, reversible, and benign condition accompanied by a pleasant affect. In contrast, HPPD is a generally long-term, distressing, spontaneous, recurrent, pervasive, either slowly reversible or irreversible, nonbenign condition accompanied by an unpleasant dysphoric affect.[55] In most cases, most HPPD cases have been induced by LSD or PCP.[56]

Additional long-term effects were associated with thinning of the posterior cingulate cortex, thickening of the anterior cingulate cortex, and decreased neocortical 5-HT2A receptor binding. These results suggest that hallucinogens increase introspection and positive mood by modulating brain activity in the fronto-temporo-parieto-occipital cortex.[57]

At very high doses, patients have experienced severe behavioral disorders, paranoid ideations, and amnesia for the entire period of the in-hospital stay. In addition, shallow respiratory excursions and periods of apnea and cyanosis coincided with generalized extensor spasm and spasm of neck muscles. In drug-abusing patients,

PCP toxic psychosis should be considered if patients present with schizophrenia-like symptoms, psychosis, or other bizarre behavior, whether they admit to taking PCP or not.[58]

It is estimated that 10.2% of the current US population has taken LSD. That averages to approximately 31 million people that have ever used LSD. Thus far, there has not been a single documented death owing to LSD at recreational doses. When fatalities occur after LSD use, they have been attributed to risky and dangerous activities, such as walking across a busy highway, attempting to swim, or rock climbing. In the only 2 documented cases when LSD presumably directly led to fatality, postmortem analysis indicated that the decedents had ingested massive doses of LSD.[59]

TREATMENT OPTIONS

For hallucinogen use disorder and substance-induced psychosis, no controlled trials for treatment have been performed. No established pharmacologic treatments to decrease use of hallucinogens currently exist. Medication options are often used to control the behavioral symptoms.

SUMMARY

Even though hallucinogens have been around for a millennium, there are limited data showing their impact in older adults. However, it is known that when these substances are used, they can induce a variety of effects, including hallucinations, depersonalization, and derealization as well as changes in one's mood and behaviors. The effects may last for a short period or even cause long-term issues. Hallucinogens are not usually associated with dependency and uncontrollable drug-seeking behaviors. Therefore, there has been a renewed interest in possible therapeutic benefits, notably at small doses. More time and in-depth studies are needed in humans across all ages before we can truly gain more insight into the actual benefits versus long-term consequences of these powerful, mind-altering agents, notably in the geriatric population.

CLINICS CARE POINTS

- Hallucinogens are a diverse group of drugs that alter perception, thoughts, and feelings. They cause hallucinations or sensations and images that seem real, but they are not.
- Hallucinogens are split into 2 categories: classical hallucinogens and dissociative drugs.
- They produce their psychedelic effect via their agonistic action on 5-HT2A receptors, independently from dopamine stimulation.
- These substances are not usually viewed as drugs of abuse because of a lack of dependency or dopamine reward.
- Some long-term consequences associated with their use include flashbacks and hallucinogen persisting perception disorder.
- Hallucinogens may have potential therapeutic benefits to enhance mood, decrease anxiety, and decrease posttraumatic stress disorder, help with alcohol use disorder, and promote neuroplasticity.

DISCLOSURE

The authors have nothing to disclose.

REFERENCES

1. Lewin L. Phantastica, narcotic and stimulating drugs: their use and abuse. JAMA 1932;98(16):1403.
2. Nichols DE. Psychedelics [published correction appears in Pharmacol Rev. 2016 Apr;68(2):356]. Pharmacol Rev 2016;68(2):264–355.
3. Johnson MW, Griffiths RR. Potential therapeutic effects of psilocybin. Neurotherapeutics 2017;14(3):734–40.
4. Carhart-Harris RL, Roseman L, Bolstridge M, et al. Psilocybin for treatment-resistant depression: fMRI-measured brain mechanisms. Sci Rep 2017;7(1):13187.
5. Krebs TS, Johansen PØ. Lysergic acid diethylamide (LSD) for alcoholism: meta-analysis of randomized controlled trials. J Psychopharmacol 2012;26(7):994–1002.
6. Berman RM, Cappiello A, Anand A, et al. Antidepressant effects of ketamine in depressed patients. Biol Psychiatry 2000;47(4):351–4.
7. Cassels BK, Sáez-Briones P. Dark classics in chemical neuroscience: mescaline. ACS Chem Neurosci 2018;9(10):2448–58.
8. Carod-Artal FJ. Hallucinogenic drugs in pre-Columbian Mesoamerican cultures. Neurologia 2015;30(1):42–9.
9. Fantegrossi WE, Murnane KS, Reissig CJ. The behavioral pharmacology of hallucinogens. Biochem Pharmacol 2008;75(1):17–33.
10. Glennon RA. Neurobiology of hallucinogens. In: Galanter M, Kleber H, editors. The American psychiatric publishing textbook of substance abuse treatment. 4th edition. Washington, DC: APPI; 2008. p. 181–9.
11. Geyer MA, Nichols DE, Vollenweider FX. In: Squire LR, editor. Encyclopedia of neuroscience. Oxford: Academic Press; 2009. p. 741–8.
12. Hofmann A. How LSD originated. J Psychedelic Drugs 1979;11(1–2):53–60.
13. National Institute on Drug Abuse; National Institutes of Health; U.S. Department of Health and Human Services. Hallucinogens: Drug Facts; 2019.
14. Chi T, Gold JA. A review of emerging therapeutic potential of psychedelic drugs in the treatment of psychiatric illnesses. J Neurol Sci 2020;411:116715.
15. Gabay M. The federal controlled substances act: schedules and pharmacy registration. Hosp Pharm 2013;48(6):473–4.
16. Grant BF, Saha TD, Ruan WJ, et al. Epidemiology of DSM-5 drug use disorder: results from the national epidemiologic survey on alcohol and related conditions-III. JAMA Psychiatry 2016;73(1):39–47.
17. Krebs TS, Johansen PØ. Over 30 million psychedelic users in the United States. F1000Res 2013;2:98.
18. Shalit N, Rehm J, Lev-Ran S. Epidemiology of hallucinogen use in the U.S. results from the National Epidemiologic Survey on alcohol and related conditions III. Addict Behav 2019;89:35–43.
19. Yockey RA, Vidourek RA, King KA. Trends in LSD use among US adults: 2015-2018. Drug Alcohol Depend 2020;212:108071.
20. Sadzot B, Baraban JM, Glennon RA, et al. Hallucinogenic drug interactions at human brain 5-HT2 receptors: implications for treating LSD-induced hallucinogenesis. Psychopharmacology (Berl) 1989;98(4):495–9.
21. Vollenweider FX, Vollenweider-Scherpenhuyzen MF, Bäbler A, et al. Psilocybin induces schizophrenia-like psychosis in humans via a serotonin-2 agonist action. Neuroreport 1998;9(17):3897–902.

22. Lodge D, Mercier MS. Ketamine and phencyclidine: the good, the bad and the unexpected. Br J Pharmacol 2015;172(17):4254–76.
23. Nichols DE. Hallucinogens. Pharmacol Ther 2004;101(2):131–81.
24. Lyvers M, Meester M. Illicit use of LSD or psilocybin, but not MDMA or nonpsychedelic drugs, is associated with mystical experiences in a dose-dependent manner. J Psychoactive Drugs 2012;44(5):410–7.
25. Family N, Maillet EL, Williams LTJ, et al. Safety, tolerability, pharmacokinetics, and pharmacodynamics of low dose lysergic acid diethylamide (LSD) in healthy older volunteers. Psychopharmacology (Berl) 2020;237(3):841–53.
26. Schmid Y, Enzler F, Gasser P, et al. Acute effects of lysergic acid diethylamide in healthy subjects. Biol Psychiatry 2015;78(8):544–53.
27. Hollister LE. Effects of hallucinogens in humans. In: Jacob BL, editor. Hallucinogens: neurochemical, behavioral, and clinical perspectives. New York: Raven Press; 1984. p. 19–33.
28. Johnson M, Richards W, Griffiths R. Human hallucinogen research: guidelines for safety. J Psychopharmacol 2008;22(6):603–20.
29. Hwang KAJ, Saadabadi A. Lysergic acid diethylamide (LSD). In: StatPearls. Treasure Island (FL): StatPearls Publishing; 2020.
30. Anderson T, Petranker R, Christopher A, et al. Psychedelic microdosing benefits and challenges: an empirical codebook. Harm Reduct J 2019;16(1):43.
31. Hutten NRPW, Mason NL, Dolder PC, et al. Motives and side-effects of microdosing with psychedelics among users. Int J Neuropsychopharmacol 2019;22(7): 426–34.
32. Carhart-Harris RL, Leech R, Williams TM, et al. Implications for psychedelic-assisted psychotherapy: functional magnetic resonance imaging study with psilocybin. Br J Psychiatry 2012;200(3):238–44.
33. Kraehenmann R, Preller KH, Scheidegger M, et al. Psilocybin-induced decrease in amygdala reactivity correlates with enhanced positive mood in healthy volunteers. Biol Psychiatry 2015;78(8):572–81.
34. Ross S, Bossis A, Guss J, et al. Rapid and sustained symptom reduction following psilocybin treatment for anxiety and depression in patients with life-threatening cancer: a randomized controlled trial. J Psychopharmacol 2016; 30(12):1165–80.
35. Bershad AK, Preller KH, Lee R, et al. Preliminary report on the effects of a low dose of LSD on resting-state amygdala functional connectivity. Biol Psychiatry Cogn Neurosci Neuroimaging 2020;5(4):461–7.
36. Hendricks PS, Thorne CB, Clark CB, et al. Classic psychedelic use is associated with reduced psychological distress and suicidality in the United States adult population. J Psychopharmacol 2015;29(3):280–8.
37. George D, Gálvez V, Martin D, et al. Pilot randomized controlled trial of titrated subcutaneous ketamine in older patients with treatment-resistant depression. Am J Geriatr Psychiatry 2017;25(11):1199–209.
38. Bryant KA, Altinay M, Finnegan N, et al. Effects of repeated intravenous ketamine in treatment-resistant geriatric depression: a case series. J Clin Psychopharmacol 2019;39(2):158–61.
39. Corriger A, Pickering G. Ketamine and depression: a narrative review. Drug Des Devel Ther 2019;13:3051–67.
40. Ochs-Ross R, Daly EJ, Zhang Y, et al. Efficacy and safety of esketamine nasal spray plus an oral antidepressant in elderly patients with treatment-resistant depression-TRANSFORM-3. Am J Geriatr Psychiatry 2020;28(2):121–41.

41. Palhano-Fontes F, Barreto D, Onias H, et al. Rapid antidepressant effects of the psychedelic ayahuasca in treatment-resistant depression: a randomized placebo-controlled trial. Psychol Med 2019;49(4):655–63.

42. Moreno FA, Wiegand CB, Taitano EK, et al. Safety, tolerability, and efficacy of psilocybin in 9 patients with obsessive-compulsive disorder. J Clin Psychiatry 2006; 67(11):1735–40.

43. Mithoefer MC, Wagner MT, Mithoefer AT, et al. The safety and efficacy of {+/-}3,4-methylenedioxymethamphetamine-assisted psychotherapy in subjects with chronic, treatment-resistant posttraumatic stress disorder: the first randomized controlled pilot study [published correction appears in J Psychopharmacol. 2011 Jun;25(6):852]. J Psychopharmacol 2011;25(4):439–52.

44. Bogenschutz MP, Forcehimes AA, Pommy JA, et al. Psilocybin-assisted treatment for alcohol dependence: a proof-of-concept study. J Psychopharmacol 2015; 29(3):289–99.

45. Johnson MW, Garcia-Romeu A, Cosimano MP, et al. Pilot study of the 5-HT2AR agonist psilocybin in the treatment of tobacco addiction. J Psychopharmacol 2014;28(11):983–92.

46. Aday Js, Bloesch EK, Davoli CC. Can psychedelic drugs attenuate age-related changes in cognition and affect? J Cogn Enhanc 2020;4:219–27.

47. Tagliazucchi E, Roseman L, Kaelen M, et al. Increased global functional connectivity correlates with LSD-induced ego dissolution. Curr Biol 2016;26(8):1043–50.

48. Flanagan TW, Nichols CD. Psychedelics as anti-inflammatory agents. Int Rev Psychiatry 2018;30(4):363–75.

49. Diana CD. Silo pharma plans phase 2B trial testing low-dose psychedelics in Parkinson's. Parkinson's News Today; 2020. Available at: https://parkinsonsnewstoday.com/2020/12/04/silo-pharma-plans-phase-2b-trial-of-psychedelics-in-parkinsons/.

50. American Psychiatric Association. Diagnostic and Statistical Manual of Mental Disorders. 5th ed. Washington D.C.: 2013. http://dx.doi.org/10.1176/appi.books.9780890425596.

51. Krebs TS, Johansen P-Ø. Psychedelics and mental health: a population study. PLoS One 2013;8(8):e63972.

52. Aday JS, Mitzkovitz CM, Bloesch EK, et al. Long-term effects of psychedelic drugs: a systematic review. Neurosci Biobehav Rev 2020;113:179–89.

53. Abraham HD, Aldridge AM. Adverse consequences of lysergic acid diethylamide. Addiction 1993;88(10):1327–34.

54. Montoya AG, Sorrentino R, Lukas SE, et al. Long-term neuropsychiatric consequences of "ecstasy" (MDMA): a review. Harv Rev Psychiatry 2002;10:212–20.

55. Lerner AG, Gelkopf M, Skladman I, et al. Flashback and hallucinogen persisting perception disorder: clinical aspects and pharmacological treatment approach. Isr J Psychiatry Relat Sci 2002;39:92–9.

56. Martinotti G, Santacroce R, Pettorruso M, et al. Hallucinogen persisting perception disorder: etiology, clinical features, and therapeutic perspectives. Brain Sci 2018;8(3):47.

57. Dos Santos RG, Bouso JC, Alcázar-Córcoles MÁ, et al. Efficacy, tolerability, and safety of serotonergic psychedelics for the management of mood, anxiety, and substance-use disorders: a systematic review of systematic reviews. Expert Rev Clin Pharmacol 2018;11(9):889–902.

58. Jacob MS, Carlen PL, Marshman JA, et al. Phencyclidine ingestion: drug abuse and psychosis. Int J Addict 1981;16(4):749–58.

59. Nichols DE. Dark classics in chemical neuroscience: lysergic acid diethylamide (LSD). ACS Chem Neurosci 2018;9(10):2331–43.

Cannabis Use and Misuse in Older Adults

Rita Khoury, MD[a,b,c,*], Peter Maliha, MD[a,b], Roy Ibrahim, BS[b]

KEYWORDS

- Cannabis • Elderly • Disorder • Marijuana • Medical • Misuse • Recreational • Use

KEY POINTS

- Between 2015 and 2018, there was a 75% relative increase in the prevalence of past-year cannabis use among American adults aged 65 years and older, with 2.7 million engaging in past-year cannabis use.
- Population aging, legalization of medical and/or recreational cannabis, and more lenient perceptions of seniors toward cannabis use may have contributed to a surge in the prevalence of cannabis use and use disorder in this population.
- Evidence regarding the efficacy of cannabis for treating medical conditions, such as nausea, insomnia, chronic pain, and neuropsychiatric symptoms in dementia, is still lacking. Cannabis use in seniors is associated with increased cardiovascular risk, pulmonary and gastrointestinal diseases, problematic drug-drug interaction, sedation, dizziness, cognitive impairment (including impaired driving), and other neuropsychiatric disorders, such as depression, anxiety, suicidality, and psychosis.
- Physicians are recommended to inform their older patients about the balance benefits/risks associated with use, and systematically screen for patterns of use, and possible misuse.
- More research is needed to determine optimal and safe doses and formulations of THC/CBD to be used, in addition to adapting and validating appropriate screening tools for detection of cannabis use disorder in older adults.

INTRODUCTION

Cannabis use among individuals aged 50 years and older is on an unprecedented rise.[1] Cannabis is the most frequently used illegal psychoactive substance by older adults.[2]

[a] Department of Psychiatry and Clinical Psychology, Saint Georges Hospital University Medical Center, Beirut, Lebanon; [b] Faculty of Medicine, University of Balamand, Beirut, Lebanon; [c] Department of Psychiatry and Behavioral Neurosciences, Saint Louis University School of Medicine, St Louis, MO, USA
* Corresponding author. Department of Psychiatry and Clinical Psychology, Saint Georges Hospital University Medical Center, Youssef Sursock Street, PO Box 166378, Beirut, Lebanon.
E-mail address: rita.khoury@idraac.org

Clin Geriatr Med 38 (2022) 67–83
https://doi.org/10.1016/j.cger.2021.07.003
0749-0690/22/© 2021 Elsevier Inc. All rights reserved.

Cannabis, also known as marijuana, is a plant that is composed of more than 500 components, of which the Delta-9-tetrahydro-cannabinol (THC) and cannabidiol (CBD) are extensively studied in the literature. The major physiologic effects of cannabinoids are mediated by 2 G-protein coupled receptors named cannabinoid receptor 1 (CB1R) and cannabinoid receptor 2 (CB2R). CB1R distribution spans the entire central nervous system, with prominence in the cortex, hippocampus, amygdala, basal ganglia, and cerebellum. CB1R is also expressed peripherally in the thyroid and adrenal glands, adipocytes, and gastrointestinal tract.[3] CB2R is mainly expressed in the immune system and hematopoietic cells. It is also expressed in the brain, but to a far lesser extent, and its role in the endocannabinoid system remains relatively unknown.[4]

THC is the primary psychoactive component that is responsible for the drug's potency, as well as side effects via its CB1R agonism. CBD binds weakly to CB1Rs and may even interfere with the binding of THC, resulting in a lack of euphoric and reinforcing effect. CBD has more selective affinity for CB2Rs that carry neuroprotective properties.[5]

In the past 2 decades, there has been an increase in the THC:CBD ratio on the cannabis market, leading to detrimental consequences on physical and mental health of consumers.[6]

Furthermore, synthetic cannabinoids, such as spice and K2, initially prepared to study the therapeutic effects of cannabis, were quickly misused: they are cheaper, and more potent and toxic than THC/natural cannabis, and go undetectable in routine drug screens, posing a significant public health concern.[7]

From medical and regulatory perspectives, the US Food and Drug Administration (FDA) has approved 3 cannabinoids drugs[8]: cannabidiol (CBD), an oral solution for the treatment of seizures in 2 rare forms of epilepsy; dronabinol (synthetic THC) to treat refractory chemotherapy-associated nausea/vomiting and human immunodeficiency virus (HIV)-related anorexia/weight loss; and nabilone (synthetic chemical structure similar to THC) for refractory chemotherapy-associated nausea/vomiting. Nabiximols, a fixed dose combination of THC and CBD (2.7 mg/2.5 mg), is an oro-mucosal spray approved by health Canada for the treatment of multiple sclerosis–related spasticity.[9] Besides these approved products, medical cannabis provided by dispensaries for several medical and neuropsychiatric conditions comes in various formulations and has unstandardized THC and CBD content. In other words, medical cannabis and recreational cannabis are not meaningfully distinct terms from a pharmacologic perspective.[10]

As the world shifts toward legalization and/or medicalization of many forms of cannabis, and as the older adults' perceptions of cannabis have become more lenient, it has become highly important to explore in depth the benefits and harms associated with cannabis increasingly used by older adults. Assessment tools to screen for cannabis use disorder in this population are discussed, in addition to management strategies.

LEGALIZATION/DECRIMINALIZATION OF CANNABIS USE

Legalization of cannabis is the process of removing all legal prohibitions against it. Cannabis would then be available to the adult general population (>21 years) for purchase and use at will, like tobacco and alcohol. Decriminalization is the act of removing criminal sanctions against an act, article, or behavior, meaning it would remain illegal, but the legal system would not prosecute a person for possession under a specified amount.[11]

Enormous efforts were put since the late 1960s to decriminalize and legalize medicinal and/or recreational use of cannabis around the world. Uruguay, followed by Canada, were the first nations to legalize the recreational use of cannabis. In the United States, this process began with legalizing medicinal cannabis supplied by certified dispensaries in 36 states and the District of Columbia. Recreational use of cannabis has also become legal in 16 states and the District of Columbia, as of April 2021.[12] Also, 46 states legalized cannabidiol (CBD) oil for therapeutic and/or recreational use.[13]

Several studies have consistently demonstrated a correlation between the legalization of medical and/or recreational cannabis, a subsequent increased availability of the drug, and significant increases in cannabis use and cannabis use disorder.[14,15] American older adults had a significant increase in cannabis use after medical marijuana legalization, as demonstrated by a 2016 cross-sectional study that analyzed data from the National Survey of Drug Use and Health (NSDUH) between 2004 and 2013[16]: past-month cannabis use increased from 4.5% to 6.0% ($P<.0001$) in the 40 to 64 years age bracket and from 0.3% to 0.8% ($P = .0006$) in the older than 65 years population.

PREVALENCE OF CANNABIS USE/MISUSE IN OLDER ADULTS

Older adults represent the fastest growing bracket of cannabis users of any age group. There are likely several contributing factors to this growth, including recent legalization and decriminalization efforts, as well as the current geriatric population being the former young adult population from the 1970s and 1980s when cannabis was popularized within the counterculture.[17]

In the United States, there was a significant increase in the prevalence of past-year cannabis use among those older than 50 between 2006 and 2007 and 2012 to 2013: a 57.8% relative increase in use for adults aged 50 to 64 years ($P<.001$) and a 250% relative increase in use for those 65 years and older ($P = .002$).[18] Between 2015 and 2018, there was a 75% relative increase in the prevalence of past-year cannabis use among adults 65 years and older, with a sharp jump from 2.4% to 4.2% ($P = .001$).[19] In 2019, approximately 2.7 million American adults 65 and older (5.1%) engaged in past-year cannabis use.[20]

Older adults (50 years or older) represented approximately 30% and 17% of medical and nonmedical cannabis users, respectively. Medical cannabis users were more likely than nonmedical cannabis users to have a cannabis use disorder, according to the 2012 to 2013 National Epidemiologic Survey on Alcohol and Related Conditions (NESARC).[21] From 2013 to 2014, the 12-month prevalence of medical cannabis use among US adults ages 50 and older was only 0.6%.[22]

In Canada, data show that the proportion of older cannabis users has been steadily growing, whereas that of young users has been relatively shrinking. In 1977, users aged 18 to 29 years represented 82% of the past-year cannabis use population, decreasing to 51% in 2015, while the population aged 30 to 49 increased from 15% to 26%, and the population aged 50 years and older increased approximately 700% from 3% to 23% during this time period.[23]

PERCEPTIONS OF SENIORS REGARDING CANNABIS USE

In parallel with the legalization of cannabis, there has been a drastic change in the perceptions of older adults regarding the risks associated with cannabis use.

Based on data derived from the 2013 to 2015 NSDUH involving 24,057 respondents aged 50 years and older, former and past-year cannabis users were found to have lower odds of high-risk perceptions related to cannabis, compared with never-users. More frequent cannabis use among past-year users was associated with a lower likelihood to have high-risk perceptions (adjusted odds ratio [OR] of 0.14, 95% confidence interval [CI] 0.07–0.28 for >300 days compared with 1–11 days of cannabis use). However, those who had cannabis use disorder according to the *Diagnostic and Statistical Manual of Mental Disorders, Fifth Edition* (DSM-5) criteria were 3.5 times more likely to perceive high risks related to cannabis use.[24]

In 2 qualitative studies, American older cannabis users found this drug to be safer and more effective than prescription drugs to treat several medical conditions, including chronic pain.[25,26] Many of these patients identified lack of physicians' support and knowledge in this specialized field as barriers for them to get medicinal cannabis.[26]

More recently, 2 scales composed of 12 items each were developed to assess attitudes of adults 60 years and older toward the use of medical and recreational cannabis, within 3 dimensions (affective, cognitive, and social perception).[27] Interestingly, this study demonstrated initial evidence about the incongruence in attitudes toward medical and recreational cannabis: although 60% of older participants strongly agreed that "use of medical cannabis is acceptable," only about 30% strongly agreed with the acceptability of recreational cannabis. Approximately 60% were in favor of legalizing medical cannabis, less than 30% agreed on this statement for recreational cannabis. A great proportion of older adults perceived recreational cannabis as more risky and a potential gateway drug, in comparison with medical cannabis.[27] These adapted scales will help researchers and health care workers better understand the perceptions of seniors and design tailored prevention and treatment strategies for this population.

ROUTES OF ADMINISTRATION IN OLDER ADULTS

Historically, smoking cannabis (primarily via rolled joint/blunt and pipe/bong) has been the predominant route of administration across all ages: in 2014, the analysis of a large-scale US survey including more than 4000 participants showed that 92.1% of the sample used cannabis via combustion only (95% CI 86.7%–95.4%).[28] However, with the widespread cannabis legalization and decriminalization, other formulations are becoming increasingly popular. They include inhalation of vaporized dried flowers or cannabis oil ("vaping") and orally ingesting edible products ("edibles").[29]

In 2015, a cross-sectional study on baby boomer cannabis users (n = 97, median age 58 years) showed that recreational users were more likely to adopt combustion as their primary delivery system over medical users (94% vs 75%, respectively). Ingestion of cannabis was preferred by medical cannabis users over recreational users (12.5% vs 3% respectively). Medical cannabis users were 5 times more likely to use a combination of intake methods compared with recreational users (9.3% vs 1.5%). These results indicate that legalization of medical cannabis via dispensaries offered several routes of administration options for medical cannabis users.[30] Haug and colleagues[31] also explored the preferred route of administration by age groups in a sample of 217 participants (median age: 41.2) using medical marijuana in San Francisco, California, in 2017. Older adults were significantly more likely to ingest cannabis compared with younger adults (25% vs 7% respectively, $P = .021$).

ADVERSE EFFECTS OF CANNABIS IN OLDER ADULTS

Older adults undergo several age-related changes that may trigger or accentuate the deleterious effects of cannabis on their physical and mental health, as shown in **Table 1**.

Table 1	
Adverse effects of cannabis use in older adults	
Cardiovascular	Hypertension/hypotension; coronary artery disease, arrhythmias; cerebrovascular accidents, myocardial infarction, cardiac arrest
Pulmonary	Cough, phlegm production, wheezing, altered pulmonary function tests, chronic obstructive pulmonary disease, spontaneous pneumothorax, bullous emphysema
Gastrointestinal	Gastric and colonic dysmotility, appetite modifications (suppression/stimulation), cannabis hyperemesis syndrome Diarrhea (with CBD)
Drug-drug interaction	Polypharmacy; THC: CYP1A2 inducer; CBD: CYP1A2, 2D6, 3A4 inhibitor
Central nervous system	Dizziness, sedation, cognitive impairment, impaired driving
Psychiatric	Mood disorders (major depressive disorder, dysthymia, bipolar disorder)/suicidality Anxiety disorders/posttraumatic stress disorder Psychotic disorders Alcohol and other substance use disorders
Risk for elder abuse	Notably in those with cognitive impairment

Abbreviations: CBD, cannabidiol; CYP, cytochrome; THC, Delta-9-tetrahydro-cannabinol.

Cardiovascular System

Low doses of cannabis stimulate the sympathetic system, leading to hypertension and tachycardia, whereas higher doses stimulate the parasympathetic system, leading to hypotension and bradycardia. Orthostatic hypotension is associated with increased risk of falls, which is problematic in older adults. In addition, cannabis is associated with decreased cerebral blood velocity, leading to an increased risk of ischemic stroke. It can also adversely affect the myocardial oxygen supply and demand, increasing the risk of myocardial infarction. Increased thrombotic risk is also exacerbated by platelet activation, leading to a procoagulant state.[32,33] Furthermore, cannabis smoke is associated with oxidant damage, inflammation, endothelial dysfunction, and induction of a prothrombotic state resulting in an increased risk of acute coronary syndrome, stroke, and sudden cardiac death.[34] Cardiac arrythmias and palpitations have also been reported, the most common one being atrial fibrillation, followed by ventricular fibrillation. These cases are linked to the sympathetic activation and catecholamine release, induced by cannabis use.[32,33] Thus, the American Heart Association issued in 2020 a position statement urging caution in use of medical cannabis in older adults due to possible detrimental cardiovascular effects.[35]

Respiratory

Cannabis use has been associated with an increase in airway resistance and hyperinflation, leading to coughing and impaired pulmonary functions. These effects vary depending on the dose, potency, and route of administration of cannabis.[36]

A systematic review on the effects of inhalational cannabis on the respiratory system showed a significant association with spontaneous pneumothorax, bullous emphysema, or chronic obstructive pulmonary disease (COPD). Other commonly reported symptoms include wheezing, shortness of breath, altered pulmonary function tests, cough, and phlegm production.[37]

Gastrointestinal

In vitro studies involving human and animal tissues have demonstrated cannabinoids to impact intestinal motility. Human studies involving dronabinol administered orally have shown delay in gastric emptying and colonic transit.[38] Prolonged gastric emptying is associated with early satiety and may serve as a weight loss, contrary to the well-known neurologically mediated appetite stimulation and nausea suppression effect induced by cannabis.[39] Another infrequent but severe adverse gastrointestinal event associated with chronic cannabis use is cannabinoid hyperemesis syndrome. It is characterized by a cyclical pattern (every few weeks or months) of nausea, vomiting, and abdominal pain after using cannabis, following several years of cannabis use, resulting in chronic overstimulation of cannabinoid receptors. It may go undetected in older adults and may be mistaken for acute coronary disease or a gastrointestinal infection.[40]

CBD alone has also been shown to be associated with a significant increased risk of inducing diarrhea (OR 5.03; 95% CI 1.44–17.61), compared with placebo, in a recent systematic review involving 12 randomized controlled trials.[41] This is particularly concerning in older adults because of the increased risk of dehydration, electrolyte disturbances, and delirium.

Central Nervous System

The most common adverse events reported with medical cannabis in older adults include dizziness, drowsiness, and sedation.[42,43] This is particularly concerning given the increased risk of falls in older adults.

Neuropsychiatric Side Effects

Affective, psychotic disorders and suicide

Choi and colleagues[44] demonstrated that users of cannabis as the only illicit drug had a higher likelihood of developing lifetime and past-year major depressive disorder (MDD), when compared with nonusers (OR 1.73; 95% CI 1.36–2.20, and OR 1.54; 95% CI 1.17–2.03, respectively). The odds of developing lifetime and past-year MDD further increased when cannabis was used alongside other illicit drugs (OR 2.50; 95% CI 1.66–3.76, and OR 2.75; 95% CI 1.75–4.33, respectively).[44] Past-year cannabis users reported lifetime and past-year depression rates of 32.3% and 17.33%, respectively.[45,46]

Other affective disorders precipitated by cannabis use in older adults include dysthymia reaching 14% of past-year users compared with 4.21% of never-users. Past-year and lifetime prevalence rates of bipolar disorder among this older population range between 3.82% (vs 0.89% among nonusers; $P<.001$) and 4.25% (vs 1.45% among nonusers; $P<.001$), respectively.[47]

Polydrug use (cannabis and other illicit drugs) was found to be associated with increased risk (OR 2.44; 95% CI 1.58–3.77) of suicidal thoughts (reaching 13%) compared with no use (2.2%; $P<.001$) among adults aged 50 years and older. Particularly in those who suffer from MDD, cannabis use frequency was correlated with the emergence of suicidal ideations.[44] Lifetime suicidal attempts were also more likely to occur in older cannabis users than older nonusers.[46]

Cannabis use is also associated with increased risk of psychosis, up to 40% from baseline. This risk can increase up to 200% in young adults with heavy consumption.[48] Data in older adults is, however, lacking.

Anxiety, trauma-related disorders, and substance use disorders

Anxiety is a common reason for older adults to use cannabis. In a sample of 82 older cannabis users living in California, 25% reported using it to relieve their anxiety.[49] In a large cross-sectional study analyzing data from the 2012 to 2013 NESARC, approximately 23% of past-year cannabis users aged 50 years and older reported a past-year diagnosis of anxiety disorders, whereas approximately 30% reported a lifetime diagnosis of anxiety disorders, including specific phobia, social phobia, panic disorder, agoraphobia, or generalized anxiety disorder.[46] In addition, past-year cannabis users reported significantly more past-year posttraumatic stress disorder (PTSD) (9.44% vs 3.20% in never-users) and lifetime PTSD (11.57% vs 4.08% in never-users); $P<.001$ for both. All diagnoses were made according to the DSM-5 criteria.[46]

Within the same study, a significant proportion of older cannabis users were found to be polysubstance users: 8.4% of past-year cannabis users had other drug use disorders, 29.3% had alcohol use disorder, and 47.5% had tobacco/nicotine use disorder. Among never-users, the corresponding rates were 0.67%, 6.3%, and 15.6%, respectively. Also, 17.5% of past-year cannabis users had past-year cannabis use disorder.[46]

Cognitive impairment

In terms of cognitive functioning, the memory domain is predominantly affected by cannabis use.[50] The impact of cannabis on the brain is closely correlated with the frequency and duration of use.[50,51] Using data from the NESARC, self-reported cognitive function was investigated among older cannabis users, using the Executive Function Index. Current users, particularly those with cannabis use disorder, reported worse cognition than never or former users. Among both former and current users, greater duration of past use was associated with worse cognition. Frequent use within the past 12 months was associated with worse cognition among current users, but daily users reported better cognition compared with monthly or weekly users. This finding may be explained by the fact that heavy drug use (daily) may impair meta-cognition (awareness of deficits), and highlights the need for neuropsychological testing for an objective assessment in those instances rather than relying on self-report.[52]

From a structural perspective, cannabis use was found to be associated with gray matter volume reduction in the medial temporal cortex, temporal pole, parahippocampal gyrus, insula, and orbitofrontal cortex. These regions rich in CB1Rs are functionally associated with motivational, emotional, and affective processing. Most importantly, a decrease in gray matter volume can occur with a heavy amount of cannabis consumption, independent of age of onset of use.[53]

Cognitive impairment, whether associated with acute intoxication or chronic cannabis use, is also reflected by impaired driving and consequent motor vehicle accidents. Using data from the 2013 to 2014 NSDUH, one-third of past-year cannabis users aged 50 years and older reported past-year driving under the influence. Those with cannabis use disorder were 2.6 times more likely than those without the disorder to report driving under the influence, after controlling for alcohol use disorder, other illicit drug use, and sociodemographic and health/mental health statuses.[54]

In a unique crossover randomized controlled trial, Arkell and colleagues[55] investigated the effects of vaporized 13.75 mg of THC, 13.75 mg of CBD, and 13.75 mg of THC/CBD compared with placebo on driving performance in 26 young patients, mean age 23.2 (SD = 2.6) years. The primary outcome was the SD of lateral position (SDLP; a measure of lane weaving) during 100-km, on-road driving tests that commenced at 40 minutes and 240 minutes after cannabis consumption. After 40 to 100 minutes, SDLP was significantly increased by THC-dominant cannabis and THC/CBD-equivalent cannabis but not by CBD-dominant cannabis, relative to placebo; 8.5% of the driving tests were terminated because of safety concerns.[55] Although this study was conducted in young adults, it sheds light on the immediate

Table 2
Medications metabolized by CYP450 enzymes in relation with THC/CBD

CYP	Drug Substrates
CYP1A2	Acetaminophen Asenapine Caffeine Clozapine Duloxetine Haloperidol Mirtazapine Ondansetron Ropinirole Olanzapine Theophylline
CYP3A4	Amlodipine Atorvastatin Buspirone Clarithromycin Carbamazepine Codeine Cyclosporin Diazepam Diltiazem Erythromycin Felodipine Haloperidol Iloperidone Lovastatin Losartan Mirtazapine Midazolam Macrolides Nifedipine Quinidine Sertraline Terfenadine Trazodone Verapamil Venlafaxine
CYP2C9	Diclofenac Losartan Valproic acid Warfarin
CYP2D6	Aripiprazole Duloxetine Fluoxetine haloperidol Imipramine Nortriptyline Paroxetine Risperidone Sertraline Venlafaxine
CYP2C19	Amitriptyline Citalopram Diazepam

(continued on next page)

Table 2 (continued)	
CYP	**Drug Substrates**
	Omeprazole
	Propranolol
	Valproic acid
	Warfarin

Abbreviations: CBD, cannabidiol; CYP, cytochrome; THC, Delta-9-tetrahydro-cannabinol.
Data from Lin JH, Lu AY. Inhibition and induction of cytochrome P450 and the clinical implications. Clinical pharmacokinetics. 1998;35(5):361-390; and English BA, Dortch M, Ereshefsky L, Jhee S. Clinically significant psychotropic drug-drug interactions in the primary care setting. Curr Psychiatry Rep. 2012;14(4):376-390.

impact of THC alone or in combination with CBD on driving performance. Older adults are already subject to several changes related to aging that affect their driving ability, such as vision impairment, muscle weakness, and dementias,[56] to which adding cannabis can have detrimental consequences.

Finally, older adults, especially those with cognitive impairment, can be subject to elder abuse and coercion to provide their medical cannabis prescription to unintended users.[57]

Polypharmacy

Older adults suffer from several chronic physical and mental health problems, with increased likelihood of polypharmacy. Drug-drug interactions are mostly pharmacokinetic by affecting drug metabolism enzymes such as hepatic cytochrome P450 (CYP450). Induction of CYP450 leads to reduced drug plasma levels, whereas inhibition of CYP450 leads to increased drug plasma levels leading to toxic effects.[58]

THC is metabolized by CYP2C9 and 3A4, and CBD is metabolized by CYP2C19 and 3A4. THC also acts as a CYP1A2 inducer and CBD as an inhibitor of CYP1A2, CYP2B6, CYP2C9, CYP2D6, and CYP3A4.[59,60] Both THC and CBD can thus lead to drug-drug interactions with several commonly used medication groups in older patients, including anticoagulants, antibiotics, anticonvulsants, antidepressants, and antipsychotics, as shown in **Table 2**.[58,61]

THERAPEUTIC BENEFITS OF CANNABIS AMONG OLDER ADULTS

Older adults may benefit from cannabis for various symptoms that did not respond to current standard of care strategies. These symptoms include chronic pain, spasticity, nausea and vomiting, anorexia, and neuropsychiatric symptoms, such as depression, anxiety, insomnia, agitation in dementias, and others.[62] To date, positive findings regarding efficacy of cannabis in older adults stem mostly from observational trials, providing low-quality evidence for the scientific community.

In a 6-month cohort, 2736 patients older than 65 years received cannabis (mean dose 28.8 ± 14.9 g) in the form of oil and inflorescence, delivered as flowers, capsules, and cigarettes. Indications for use were chronic pain and cancer in 90% of the cases. Other indications included Parkinson disease, amyotrophic lateral sclerosis, multiple sclerosis, PTSD, and Alzheimer disease.[63] After 6 months of treatment, 93.7% of the respondents reported improvement in their condition and the reported pain levels were significantly reduced from a median of 8 on a scale of 0 to 10 to a median of 4.6. Quality of life was also significantly improved: at baseline, 79.3% of respondents defined their quality of life as either bad or very bad, whereas after the treatment,

58.6% defined their quality of life as either good or very good (P<.001); 35.1% reported a decrease in the number of drugs or their dosage and 18.1% stopped using opioid analgesics or reduced their dose. Another cohort led by the same group of investigators involved 184 patients 65 years and older who were on medical cannabis; 84.8% reported some degree of improvement of their general health. Cannabis was well tolerated by most of the patients, and it showed potential in improving pain, sleep disturbances, nausea, vomiting, Parkinson disease, PTSD, and dementia behavioral symptoms.[42]

In addition, cannabis use in a sample of 17 adults 50 years and older, with and without HIV, was shown to significantly increase total sleep time (by more than 30 minutes; P value of .046), without any effect though on sleep efficiency.[64]

A recent systematic review[43] investigating the efficacy, safety, and tolerability of medical cannabis in adults 65 years or older reported results from 5 randomized controlled trials. These studies failed to show any statistically significant impact on dyskinesia, breathlessness resulting from COPD, and chemotherapy-induced nausea and vomiting. Two studies showed a potential benefit of dronabinol (FDA-approved synthetic cannabis) for the treatment of anorexia and behavioral symptoms in dementia.

In summary, there is no or very low-quality evidence supporting the medical use of cannabis in older adults for treatment of neuropathic or other chronic pain, insomnia, and anxiety; or cancer-related anorexia, nausea, and vomiting. There is a possible nonsignificant trend toward efficacy in treating cancer pain and spasticity in neurologic diseases, as well as agitation in neurocognitive disorders.[65] However, more robust investigations are needed to ascertain the safe and effective formulations and doses for these indications.

The synthetic oral THC analogue nabilone is a partial agonist at CB1/2R that was recently studied in a phase II randomized controlled trial[66] at the doses of 1 to 2 mg in 38 institutionalized patients with moderate to severe Alzheimer disease. Nabilone was shown to significantly decrease agitation as measured by the Cohen Mansfield Agitation Inventory (CMAI) (b = −4.0 [−6.5 to −1.5], P = .003). However, these promising findings need to be corroborated in larger, more robust trials.

CANNABIS USE DISORDER: SCREENING/DIAGNOSIS

Analysis of data from the 2012 to 2013 NESARC revealed that 10.7% and 26.9% of former and past-year cannabis users respectively had lifetime cannabis use disorder. Of those with cannabis use disorder, only 21.2% and 13.7% of past-year and former users had sought help for cannabis use problems.[47]

Detection of cannabis use disorder among older users remains challenging. Cannabis use disorder is defined by the use of cannabis for at least a 1-year period, with the presence of a minimum of 2 of the DSM-5 criteria, shown in **Box 1**.[67] However, use of the DSM-5 is questionable in the geriatric population, given that the criteria related to the impact of cannabis use on fulfilling social, interpersonal roles, or performance (eg, work, school, driving) may not always apply to older adults.[20] In addition, several medical and psychiatric concomitant disorders can mask symptoms of cannabis use disorder, including withdrawal symptoms. There is thus a need to develop and validate brief and effective screening and diagnostic tools for cannabis use disorder in this population.

The Cannabis Use Disorder Identification Test (CUDIT)[68] was recommended by both the Canadian guidelines on cannabis use disorder among older adults and the American Substance Abuse and Mental Health Administration.[20,69] The CUDIT-Revised,[70] shown in **Table 3**, is a shorter 8-item tool with superior psychometric

---

Box 1
The *Diagnostic and Statistical Manual of Mental Disorders, Fifth Edition* criteria for cannabis use disorder, American Psychiatric Association (2013)

Cannabis Used in Larger Amounts and Over a Longer Period than Intended

Repeated failed efforts to discontinue or reduce the amount of cannabis used

Great amount of time is occupied acquiring, using, or recovering from the effects of cannabis

Cravings or desires to use cannabis, including intrusive thoughts and images, and dreams about cannabis, or olfactory perceptions of the smell of cannabis

Continued use of cannabis despite adverse consequences from its use, such as criminal charges, ultimatums of abandonment from spouse/partner/friends, and poor productivity

Other important activities in life, such as work, school, hygiene, and responsibility to family and friends are superseded by the desire to use cannabis

Important social, occupational, or recreational activities are reduced because of use

Cannabis is used in contexts that are potentially dangerous, such as operating a motor vehicle

Use of cannabis continues despite awareness of physical or psychological problems attributed to use, such as anergia, amotivation, chronic cough

Tolerance to cannabis, as defined by progressively larger amounts of cannabis needed to obtain the psychoactive effect experienced when use first commenced, or, noticeably reduced effect of use of the same amount of cannabis

Withdrawal, defined as the typical withdrawal syndrome associated with cannabis discontinuation and cannabis or a similar substance is used to prevent withdrawal symptoms

The severity of cannabis use disorder is determined as follows: mild in case of 2 to 3 positive criteria, moderate if 4 to 5 positive criteria, and severe in the case of 6 or more criteria being met.

Data from Deborah S. Hasin, Ph.D., Charles P. O'Brien, M.D., Ph.D., Marc Auriacombe, M.D., et al. DSM-5 Criteria for Substance Use Disorders: Recommendations and Rationale. American Journal of Psychiatry. 2013;170(8):834-851.

---

properties compared with the original version, and a sensitivity and specificity of 91% and 90% respectively, using a cutoff score of 13 over 32 points.

TREATMENT OF CANNABIS USE DISORDER IN OLDER ADULTS

Evidence-based treatments for cannabis use disorder are lacking for the general population and older adults. The National Institute on Drug Abuse recommends 3 behavioral approaches to treat cannabis use disorder, including motivational interviewing, cognitive behavioral therapy, and contingency management. Psychotherapy should be adapted for older adults: repeating information, using a slower pace, offering shorter sessions, giving information in various ways (eg, verbally, visually) to match seniors' needs in terms of physical and cognitive functioning, and using age-sensitive approaches by using structured and nonconfrontational questions have been shown to be effective strategies. In some cases, providing in-home or phone services for those without transportation is needed.[20]

Older adults should be encouraged to strengthen their social network, including friends, neighbors, family members, and religious/spiritual groups to fight loneliness and social isolation and promote recovery.[17] In addition, the role of the primary care physician, geriatrician, and/or psychiatrist is substantial in diagnosing and treating depression, anxiety, PTSD, insomnia, and chronic pain. Safe and effective options in older adults include

Table 3
The cannabis use disorder identification test, revised version (CUDIT-R)

Have You Used Any Cannabis Over the Past 6 mo?	Yes or No
1. How often do you use cannabis?	Never monthly or < 2–4 times/mo or 2–3 times/wk or ≥4 times/wk
2. How many hours were you "stoned" on a typical day when you had been using cannabis?	<1 or 1–2 or 3–4 or 5–6 or ≥7
3. How often during the past 6 mo did you find that you were not able to stop using cannabis once you had started?	Never or < monthly or monthly or weekly or daily/almost daily
4. How often during the past 6 mo did you fail to do what was normally expected from you because of using cannabis?	Never or < monthly or monthly or weekly or daily/almost daily
5. How often in the past 6 mo have you devoted a great deal of your time to getting, using, or recovering from cannabis?	Never or < monthly or monthly or weekly or daily/almost daily
6. How often do you use cannabis in situations that could be physically hazardous, such as driving, operating machinery, or caring for children?	Never or < monthly or monthly or weekly or daily/almost daily
7. How often in the past 6 mo have you had a problem with your memory or concentration after using cannabis?	Never or < monthly or monthly or weekly or daily/almost daily
8. Have you ever thought about cutting down, or stopping, your use of cannabis?	Never or Yes, but not in the past 6 mo or Yes in the past 6 mo

Items 1 to 7 are scored on a Likert scale 0 to 4; item 8 is scored 0-2-4. Total score is calculated, it ranges between 0 and 32.

Data from Adamson SJ, Kay-Lambkin FJ, Baker AL, et al. An improved brief measure of cannabis misuse: the Cannabis Use Disorders Identification Test-Revised (CUDIT-R). Drug and alcohol dependence. 2010;110(1-2):137-143.

antidepressants, such as selective serotonin reuptake inhibitors (for depression/anxiety and PTSD), selective serotonin and noradrenaline reuptake inhibitors (for depression/anxiety and pain), and mirtazapine (for depression, anxiety, and insomnia).[71]

There is no approved pharmacotherapy for cannabis use disorder. Recently, CBD has been studied in a small phase II study in young adults.[72] The primary endpoints were lower urinary 11-nor-9-carboxy-δ-9-tetrahydrocannabinol (THC-COOH):creatinine ratio, and increased days per week with abstinence from cannabis during treatment. CBD at the dosages of 400 and 800 mg daily was shown to be safe and significantly superior to placebo. However, these results were not clinically relevant, given that the days of abstinence from cannabis ranged between 0.27 to 0.48 days per week. Future trials are needed in older adults and should aim for complete abstinence rather than harm reduction in this population.[73]

SUMMARY

Cannabis use and misuse in older adults have become emerging public health problems due to population aging, legalization, and medicalization of cannabis, and more lenient perceptions of older adults regarding cannabis use and minimization of its harmful effects.

Although there is solid evidence regarding the adverse events of cannabis on most organ systems in older adults, data regarding its clinical efficacy is still very limited. The primary focus of physicians should always be the safety of the treatment, "primum non nocere."[42] It is recommended they inform patients and families about the lack of sufficient evidence regarding efficacy, as well as uncertainty regarding the formulations, and doses to be used.[65] Prescription of cannabis for an older patient may be considered only after failure of evidence-based therapies. The decision should be very personalized, on a case-by-case basis, with a thorough risk-benefit assessment and a special attention to the physical and psychiatric profile of the patient, in addition to medication review.[65]

Physicians working closely with older adults should be educated about risk factors for developing cannabis use disorder in seniors, including history of substance use disorder, depression, chronic pain, grief, social isolation, and loneliness. They should implement systematic screening for substance use, including cannabis, in their interview, in a nonjudgmental way.[69]

More research is needed to adapt and validate appropriate screening and diagnostic tools for cannabis use disorder in seniors. Large randomized controlled trials of longer duration are also required to determine the efficacy and safety of certain formulations and doses of THC/CBD to be used for various clinical indications in older adults. A tighter regulation to access medical cannabis coupled with the appropriate psychoeducation regarding the benefits/risks of cannabis use in seniors may decrease the likelihood of developing cannabis use disorder, or serious adverse events among this population.

CLINICS CARE POINTS

- Cannabis use is on the rise among older adults, notably with the medicalization/legalization of marijuina.

- There is no solid evidence supporting the use of cannabis to treat neuropsychiatric disorders or pain in older adults.

- Benefits should be weighed with risks/side effects, including cardiovascular, cognitive impairment and drug-drug interaction.

- Screening for cannabis use and misuse in older adults should be systematic among primary care physicians and geriatric practitioners.

- Cannabis misuse should be managed with psychotherapy and optimal management of primary neuropsychiatric disorders using safe and effective approved pharmacotherapy.

DISCLOSURE

The authors declare they have no disclosures.

REFERENCES

1. Colliver JD, Compton WM, Gfroerer JC, et al. Projecting drug use among aging baby boomers in 2020. Ann Epidemiol 2006;16(4):257–65.
2. Blazer DG, Wu LT. The epidemiology of substance use and disorders among middle aged and elderly community adults: national survey on drug use and health. Am J Geriatr Psychiatry 2009;17(3):237–45.

3. Zou S, Kumar U. Cannabinoid receptors and the endocannabinoid system: signaling and function in the central nervous system. Int J Mol Sci 2018; 19(3):833.

4. Atwood BK, Mackie K. CB2: a cannabinoid receptor with an identity crisis. Br J Pharmacol 2010;160(3):467–79.

5. Cohen K, Weinstein AM. Synthetic and non-synthetic cannabinoid drugs and their adverse effects-A review from public health prospective. Front Public Health 2018;6:162.

6. Lafaye G, Karila L, Blecha L, et al. Cannabis, cannabinoids, and health. Dialogues Clin Neurosci 2017;19(3):309–16.

7. Mills B, Yepes A, Nugent K. Synthetic cannabinoids. Am J Med Sci 2015;350(1): 59–62.

8. O'Connor SM, Lietzan E. The surprising reach of FDA regulation of cannabis, even after descheduling. Am Univ Law Rev 2019;68(3):823–925.

9. Nabiximols. Available at: https://go.drugbank.com/drugs/DB14011. Accessed May 30, 2021.

10. Levinsohn EA, Hill KP. Clinical uses of cannabis and cannabinoids in the United States. J Neurol Sci 2020;411:116717.

11. Svrakic DM, Lustman PJ, Mallya A, et al. Legalization, decriminalization & medicinal use of cannabis: a scientific and public health perspective. Mo Med 2012; 109(2):90–8.

12. Jeremy Berke SG, Yeji Jesse L. Marijuana legalization is sweeping the US. See every state where cannabis is legal. 2021. Available at: https://www. businessinsider.com/legal-marijuana-states-2018-1. Accessed May 30, 2021.

13. Blake D. What states legalized CBD oil: 2021 update 2021. Available at: https:// americanmarijuana.org/what-states-is-cbd-oil-legal/. Accessed May 30, 2021.

14. Wen H, Hockenberry JM, Cummings JR. The effect of medical marijuana laws on adolescent and adult use of marijuana, alcohol, and other substances. J Health Econ 2015;42:64–80.

15. Hasin DS, Sarvet AL, Cerdá M, et al. US adult illicit cannabis use, cannabis use disorder, and medical marijuana laws: 1991-1992 to 2012-2013. JAMA Psychiatry 2017;74(6):579–88.

16. Martins SS, Mauro CM, Santaella-Tenorio J, et al. State-level medical marijuana laws, marijuana use and perceived availability of marijuana among the general U.S. population. Drug Alcohol Depend 2016;169:26–32.

17. Lloyd SL, Striley CW. Marijuana use among adults 50 years or older in the 21st century. Gerontol Geriatr Med 2018;4. 2333721418781668.

18. Han BH, Sherman S, Mauro PM, et al. Demographic trends among older cannabis users in the United States, 2006-13. Addiction 2017;112(3):516–25.

19. Han BH, Palamar JJ. Marijuana use by middle-aged and older adults in the United States, 2015-2016. Drug Alcohol Depend 2018;191:374–81.

20. Substance Abuse and Mental Health Services Administration. Treating Substance Use Disorder in Older Adults. Treatment Improvement Protocol (TIP) Series No. 26, SAMHSA Publication No. PEP20-02-01-011. Rockville, MD: Substance Abuse and Mental Health Services Administration; 2020.

21. Choi NG, DiNitto DM, Marti CN. Nonmedical versus medical marijuana use among three age groups of adults: associations with mental and physical health status. Am J Addict 2017;26(7):697–706.

22. Compton WM, Han B, Hughes A, et al. Use of marijuana for medical purposes among adults in the United States. JAMA 2017;317(2):209–11.

23. Ialomiteanu AR, Hamilton HA, Adlaf EM, et al. CAMH monitor e-report: substance use, mental health and well-being among Ontario adults, 1977–2015 (CAMH research document series No. 45). Toronto, ON: Centre for Addiction and Mental Health; 2016. Available at: www.camh.ca/en/research/news_and_publications/%20Pages/camh_monitor.aspx.

24. Choi NG, DiNitto DM, Marti CN. Older marijuana users' marijuana risk perceptions: associations with marijuana use patterns and marijuana and other substance use disorders. Int Psychogeriatr 2017;30(9):1311–22.

25. Lau N, Sales P, Averill S, et al. A safer alternative: cannabis substitution as harm reduction. Drug Alcohol Rev 2015;34(6):654–9.

26. Manning L, Bouchard L. Medical cannabis use: exploring the perceptions and experiences of older adults with chronic conditions. Clin Gerontol 2021;44(1): 32–41.

27. Arora K, Qualls SH, Bobitt J, et al. Measuring attitudes toward medical and recreational cannabis among older adults in Colorado. Gerontologist 2020;60(4): e232–41.

28. Schauer GL, King BA, Bunnell RE, et al. Toking, vaping, and eating for health or fun: marijuana use patterns in adults, U.S., 2014. Am J Prev Med 2016;50(1):1–8.

29. Meacham MC, Paul MJ, Ramo DE. Understanding emerging forms of cannabis use through an online cannabis community: an analysis of relative post volume and subjective highness ratings. Drug Alcohol Depend 2018;188:364–9.

30. Murphy F, Sales P, Murphy S, et al. Baby boomers and cannabis delivery systems. J Drug Issues 2015;45(3):293–313.

31. Haug NA, Padula CB, Sottile JE, et al. Cannabis use patterns and motives: a comparison of younger, middle-aged, and older medical cannabis dispensary patients. Addict Behav 2017;72:14–20.

32. Latif Z, Garg N. The impact of marijuana on the cardiovascular system: a review of the most common cardiovascular events associated with marijuana use. J Clin Med 2020;9(6):1925.

33. Pacher P, Steffens S, Haskó G, et al. Cardiovascular effects of marijuana and synthetic cannabinoids: the good, the bad, and the ugly. Nat Rev Cardiol 2018;15(3): 151–66.

34. Benowitz NL. Managing cannabis use in patients with cardiovascular disease. Can J Cardiol 2019;35(2):138–41.

35. Page RL, Allen LA, Kloner RA, et al. Medical marijuana, recreational cannabis, and cardiovascular health: a scientific statement from the American Heart association. Circulation 2020;142(10):e131–52.

36. Howden ML, Naughton MT. Pulmonary effects of marijuana inhalation. Expert Rev Respir Med 2011;5(1):87–92.

37. Martinasek MP, McGrogan JB, Maysonet A. A systematic review of the respiratory effects of inhalational marijuana. Respir Care 2016;61(11):1543.

38. Camilleri M. Cannabinoids and gastrointestinal motility: pharmacology, clinical effects, and potential therapeutics in humans. Neurogastroenterology Motil : official J Eur Gastrointest Motil Soc 2018;30(9):e13370.

39. Cohen L, Neuman MG. Cannabis and the gastrointestinal tract. J Pharm Pharm Sci 2020;23:301–13.

40. Chu F, Cascella M. Cannabinoid hyperemesis syndrome. In: StatPearls [Internet]. Treasure Island (FL): StatPearls Publishing; 2021. Available at: https://www.ncbi.nlm.nih.gov/books/NBK549915/. Accessed May 30, 2021.

41. Chesney E, Oliver D, Green A, et al. Adverse effects of cannabidiol: a systematic review and meta-analysis of randomized clinical trials. Neuropsychopharmacology 2020;45(11):1799–806.

42. Abuhasira R, Ron A, Sikorin I, et al. Medical cannabis for older patients-treatment protocol and initial results. J Clin Med 2019;8(11):1819.

43. van den Elsen GA, Ahmed AI, Lammers M, et al. Efficacy and safety of medical cannabinoids in older subjects: a systematic review. Ageing Res Rev 2014;14: 56–64.

44. Choi NG, DiNitto DM, Marti CN, et al. Relationship between marijuana and other illicit drug use and depression/suicidal thoughts among late middle-aged and older adults. Int Psychogeriatr 2016;28(4):577–89.

45. Choi NG, DiNitto DM, Marti CN. Older marijuana users: life stressors and perceived social support. Drug Alcohol Depend 2016;169:56–63.

46. Choi NG, DiNitto DM, Marti CN. Older-adult marijuana users and ex-users: comparisons of sociodemographic characteristics and mental and substance use disorders. Drug Alcohol Depend 2016;165:94–102.

47. Choi NG, DiNitto DM, Marti CN. Older adults who use or have used marijuana: help-seeking for marijuana and other substance use problems. J Substance Abuse Treat 2017;77:185–92.

48. Moore THM, Zammit S, Lingford-Hughes A, et al. Cannabis use and risk of psychotic or affective mental health outcomes: a systematic review. Lancet 2007; 370(9584):319–28.

49. Yang K, Moore A, Nguyen K, et al. Cannabis use for anxiety among older adults. Am J Geriatr Psychiatry 2020;28(4):S81–2.

50. Broyd SJ, van Hell HH, Beale C, et al. Acute and chronic effects of cannabinoids on human cognition-A systematic review. Biol Psychiatry 2016;79(7):557–67.

51. Kelleher LM, Stough C, Sergejew AA, et al. The effects of cannabis on information-processing speed. Addict Behav 2004;29(6):1213–9.

52. Benitez A, Lauzon S, Nietert PJ, et al. Self-reported cognition and marijuana use in older adults: results from the national epidemiologic survey on alcohol and related conditions-III. Addict Behav 2020;108:106437.

53. Battistella G, Fornari E, Annoni J-M, et al. Long-term effects of cannabis on brain structure. Neuropsychopharmacology 2014;39(9):2041–8.

54. Choi NG, DiNitto DM, Marti CN. Older adults driving under the influence: associations with marijuana use, marijuana use disorder, and risk perceptions. J Appl Gerontol 2017;38(12):1687–707.

55. Arkell TR, Vinckenbosch F, Kevin RC, et al. Effect of cannabidiol and Δ9-tetrahydrocannabinol on driving performance: a randomized clinical trial. JAMA 2020; 324(21):2177–86.

56. Ikpeze TC, Elfar JC. The geriatric driver: factors that influence when to stop driving. Geriatr Orthop Surg Rehabil 2016;7(2):106–9.

57. Terry-McElrath YM, O'Malley PM, Johnston LD, et al. Diversion of medical marijuana to unintended users among U.S. adults age 35 and 55, 2013-2018. J Stud alcohol Drugs 2020;81(5):604–13.

58. Lin JH, Lu AY. Inhibition and induction of cytochrome P450 and the clinical implications. Clin Pharmacokinet 1998;35(5):361–90.

59. Alsherbiny MA, Li CG. Medicinal cannabis-potential drug interactions. Medicines (Basel) 2018;6(1):3.

60. Yamreudeewong W, Wong HK, Brausch LM, et al. Probable interaction between warfarin and marijuana smoking. Ann Pharmacother 2009;43(7–8):1347–53.

61. English BA, Dortch M, Ereshefsky L, et al. Clinically significant psychotropic drug-drug interactions in the primary care setting. Curr Psychiatry Rep 2012; 14(4):376–90.
62. Briscoe J, Casarett D. Medical marijuana use in older adults. J Am Geriatr Soc 2018;66(5):859–63.
63. Abuhasira R, Schleider LB, Mechoulam R, et al. Epidemiological characteristics, safety and efficacy of medical cannabis in the elderly. Eur J Intern Med 2018;49: 44–50.
64. Campbell LM, Tang B, Watson CW-M, et al. Cannabis use is associated with greater total sleep time in middle-aged and older adults with and without HIV: a preliminary report utilizing digital health technologies. Cannabis 2020;3(2): 180–9.
65. Minerbi A, Häuser W, Fitzcharles MA. Medical cannabis for older patients. Drugs Aging 2019;36(1):39–51.
66. Herrmann N, Ruthirakuhan M, Gallagher D, et al. Randomized placebo-controlled trial of nabilone for agitation in Alzheimer's disease. Am J Geriatr Psychiatry 2019; 27(11):1161–73.
67. Deborah SH, O'Brien CP, Auriacombe M, et al. DSM-5 criteria for substance use disorders: recommendations and rationale. Am J Psychiatry 2013;170(8):834–51.
68. Adamson SJ, Sellman JD. A prototype screening instrument for cannabis use disorder: the Cannabis Use Disorders Identification Test (CUDIT) in an alcohol-dependent clinical sample. Drug Alcohol Rev 2003;22(3):309–15.
69. Bertram JR, Porath A, Seitz D, et al. Canadian guidelines on cannabis use disorder among older adults. Can Geriatr J 2020;23(1):135–42.
70. Adamson SJ, Kay-Lambkin FJ, Baker AL, et al. An improved brief measure of cannabis misuse: the Cannabis Use Disorders Identification Test-Revised (CUDIT-R). Drug Alcohol Depend 2010;110(1–2):137–43.
71. Tham A, Jonsson U, Andersson G, et al. Efficacy and tolerability of antidepressants in people aged 65 years or older with major depressive disorder - a systematic review and a meta-analysis. J Affect Disord 2016;205:1–12.
72. Freeman TP, Hindocha C, Baio G, et al. Cannabidiol for the treatment of cannabis use disorder: a phase 2a, double-blind, placebo-controlled, randomised, adaptive Bayesian trial. Lancet Psychiatry 2020;7(10):865–74.
73. Hjorthøj C, Posselt CM, Baandrup L. Cannabidiol for cannabis use disorder: too high hopes? Lancet Psychiatry 2020;7(10):838–9.

Abuse/Misuse of Prescription Medications in Older Adults

Esra Ates Bulut, MD[a], Ahmet Turan ISIK, MD[b],*

KEYWORDS

- Inappropriate prescribing • Misuse • Abuse • Older adults • Opioids
- Benzodiazepines • Chronic pain

KEY POINTS

- With the increasing aged population, drug misuse and abuse are increasing in these patients.
- Central nervous system depressants, opioids, and stimulants are potential drugs for abuse in patients.
- Although the rate of illicit drug use is low in older adults, the rate of prescription drug abuse increases in women, those with social isolation, those with depression, and those with previous substance abuse.
- Sleep disorders (insomnia) and mental health issues, frequently reported in older patients, play an essential role in prescribing sedative and anxiolytic medications.
- Drug abuse and misuse and complications related to these conditions should be considered in the rationalization of pharmacotherapy in geriatric cases, primarily due to their preventable potential.

POLYPHARMACY AND APPROPPRIATE PRESCRIBING

Depending on developing health technologies, medications, and preventive medicine practices, life expectancy is gradually increasing, and the world population is getting older. The frequent occurrence of chronic diseases such as diabetes mellitus, coronary artery disease, hypertension, cerebrovascular disease, and neurocognitive disorders in older adults makes the use of multiple drugs (polypharmacy) an important problem in geriatric practice. Although polypharmacy is defined as "unnecessary drug use or the administration of more drugs than clinically indicated,"[1] the use of more than four drugs at the same time is generally considered to be polypharmacy

[a] Department of Geriatric Medicine, Adana City Training and Research Hospital, Adana, Turkey;
[b] Unit for Brain Aging and Dementia, Department of Geriatric Medicine, Dokuz Eylul University, School of Medicine, 35340 Balcova, IZMIR, Turkey
* Corresponding author.
E-mail address: atisik@yahoo.com

Clin Geriatr Med 38 (2022) 85–97
https://doi.org/10.1016/j.cger.2021.07.004
0749-0690/22/© 2021 Elsevier Inc. All rights reserved.

geriatric.theclinics.com

and the use of ten or more drugs at the same time as hyperpolypharmacy.[2] Even though the prevalence of polypharmacy is reported to be between 37% and 58% in community-dwelling older adults,[3] the rate reaches 80% in those staying in the nursing home.[4] Appropriate polypharmacy is defined as optimizing the treatment of patients according to the evidence in the presence of many medical diseases or in complex conditions. On the other hand, inappropriate polypharmacy is the use of multiple drugs with high risk of side effects but with low benefit from treatment.[5]

There are many factors that contribute to polypharmacy in the older adults. The adverse effects associated with these drugs play a very important role in the emergence of the condition known as the prescribing cascade, which is perceived as a new medical condition and increases the drug burden.[6] For example, for constipation, urinary retention, and abdominal pain that may develop with the use of tricyclic antidepressants, new symptomatic treatments for the side effects can be added instead of discontinuing the tricyclics. Moreover, older adults, who frequently take over-the-counter medications, vitamins, and nutritional supplements, tend not to list them when reviewing medications by health care professionals, which both increases the drug burden and causes unwanted drug interactions.[7] Pharmacokinetic and pharmacodynamic changes that develop due to aging increase the risk of adverse drug reactions. Changes occur in the distribution of drugs in the body due to metabolism in the liver, elimination in the kidneys, and changes in body composition (partial increase in adipose tissue with reduced muscle mass). However, the decrease in physiologic reserves in the organ systems in frail patients and the difficulty in the management of multiple systemic diseases easily lead to undesirable consequences.[8] Studies have shown that polypharmacy, a geriatric syndrome, is associated with the increased frequency of different geriatric syndromes such as frailty, malnutrition, gait and balance disorders, falls, cognitive impairment, depression, urinary incontinence, as well as nursing home placement, increased frequency of hospital admissions, decreased functional capacity, activities of daily living and deterioration in the quality of life, and increased health expenditures.[3,9,10] Increased age, presence of concomitant systemic diseases, cognitive impairment, psychological problems (mental health conditions), long-term care facility residency, referral to doctors in different branches (multiple subspecialists), and disabilities appear as risk factors for polypharmacy.[11] The most important risk factor is the high number of drugs prescribed.[12] Polypharmacy not only economically burdens the health care system but also reduces the patient's drug compliance and increases prescribing of potentially inappropriate medications, drug misuse, drug–drug interactions, and the risk of adverse drug events (ADEs), ADE-related hospitalization, and even mortality.[13] In a study where 27,617 elderly outpatient applications were examined in a 12-month period, it was reported that the rate of ADE was 5.5%, of which 27.6% were preventable.[14] Some drug groups, such as those often prescribed for older patients, especially those that act on the central nervous system, potentially cause more side effects. In addition to these disadvantages related to pharmacotherapy in geriatric cases, it should also be taken into account that misuse and abuse of prescription drugs are serious problems with a considerable frequency.[15] Therefore, various guidelines and scales have been developed to optimize the medical treatment of elderly patients with many complex medical conditions that are vulnerable to adverse effects of the drugs. In these scales and guidelines, drugs that are not recommended for use in the elderly, potential interactions between drugs, appropriate and inappropriate treatments according to the clinical situation are specified. Prescribing guidelines have been developed for a wide range of classes, including anticholinergic, antiparkinsonian, antispasmodic, antithrombotic, anti-infective, antidepressant, antipsychotic, sedative/hypnotic, analgesics, and cardiovascular, gastrointestinal, and genitourinary system drugs.[12] The most well-known tools in use to support appropriate prescribing in older patients are summarized in **Box 1**. It is unclear whether these tools have made clinically significant improvements in meta-analyses, but it is obvious that they reduce inappropriate prescribing.[16,17]

Drug evaluation and optimization of medical treatment is an important part of the comprehensive geriatric assessment (CGA), accepted as the gold standard, which allows for the evaluation of older adults in a holistic and patient-centered manner. It has been reported that the frequencies of polypharmacy and hyperpolypharmacy after CGA application decreased from 56% to 34% and from 12% to 3%, respectively.[2] Considering the drug groups whose frequency of use has decreased after CGA, it is noteworthy that there are antihistamines, proton pump inhibitors, non-steroidal anti-inflammatory drugs (NSAIDs), drugs initiated for dizziness, antiemetic drugs, pre-meal short-acting insulins, digoxin, benzodiazepines, antipsychotics, and anti-dementia drugs. Thus, it is shown that by discontinuing unsuitable drugs, savings of $ 153/year per capita, an expenditure of $ 67/year per capita by initiating indicated treatments, and net savings of $ 86/year per capita were provided.[2]

When prescribing in older adults, it is recommended to avoid drug groups with anticholinergic effects. Anticholinergic drug groups include bladder antispasmodics, first-generation antihistamines, tricyclic antidepressants, skeletal muscle relaxants, antiemetics, and antipsychotics.[12] Anticholinergic Drug Scale,[23] Anticholinergic Risk Scale,[24] Anticholinergic Cognitive Burden Scale,[25] and Drug Burden Index[26] to evaluate the cholinergic burden in the treatment of patients provide the opportunity to better examine the relationship between negative results that occur with exposure to anticholinergic side effects, rather than looking at individual drugs or drug classes separately. Anticholinergic effects, counted as confusion, hallucination, dry mouth, blurred vision, constipation, nausea, urinary retention, sweating, and tachycardia, pose a risk for falls, delirium, cognitive impairment, decreased physical performance, and mortality in elderly patients.[27,28]

It is necessary to prevent inappropriate polypharmacy in older patients to increase patients' adherence to treatment (ensure drugs are used at the desired dose at correct intervals to get the most benefit from medical treatment). The existence of a safer alternative to the regimen applied, adverse effects, toxicity, and the suitability of the patients to come for follow-up should be reviewed separately. Patients should be adequately informed about their medical conditions, their concerns about treatment should be eliminated, and drug use motivation should be provided. If possible, the number of daily drug doses should be minimized in terms of drug compliance by using appropriate combined preparations in which two or more drugs are used together at

---

Box 1

Assessment tools of prescribing appropriateness

American Geriatrics Society (AGS) Beers Criteria[12]

Screening Tool to Alert doctors to Right Treatment (START) and/or the Screening Tool of Older People's Prescriptions (STOPP)[18]

Fit FOR The Aged-FORTA[19]

Medication Appropriateness Index[20]

Assessing Care of Elders (ACOVE)[21]

PRISCUS List[22]

the same time.[29] In older adults with cognitive and physical disabilities and vision and hearing problems, treatment should be specifically arranged, and in some cases, the help of caregivers may be needed.

PRESCRIPTION DRUG ABUSE AND MISUSE

It has been previously stated that misuse and abuse of prescription drugs is a serious problem in older patients. Because older people are not at the forefront in social, legal, and professional areas, it is a little more difficult to notice substance and drug abuse in these people.[15] The National Institute on Drug Abuse defines drug abuse as "the intentional use of a medication without a prescription; in a way other than as prescribed; or for the experience or feeling it causes".[30] The Food and Drug Administration (FDA) describes misuse as the use of pharmaceutical medication that is, contrary to medical advice or that is, not as prescribed.[30] Misuse of medicines includes consuming extra doses, not refilling prescriptions, misunderstanding the doctor's instructions, underdosing, and taking medications at the wrong time. Chronic diseases in the older population, changes in drug metabolism, and increased potential for drug interactions make the abuse and misuse of drugs (and other substances) more dangerous than in the younger population.[31] Problems such as chronic pain in patients may make long-term use of many drugs such as opioids and NSAIDs inevitable. Therefore, although it is difficult to use drugs appropriately, economic inadequacies in these cases may increase the tendency of patients to use other patients' drugs. However, risky behaviors such as obtaining prescriptions from more than one doctor or storing medication over time are issues that should be questioned, especially in geriatric cases.[32] Thus, compliance with the treatment is negatively affected in geriatric cases, and older adults cannot benefit from the treatment effectively due to misuse. Although the rate of illicit drug use is low in the elderly, the rate of drug abuse increases in women, those with social isolation, depressives, and those who had previous substance abuse.[32] In older individuals, loss of status after retirement, decreased social support, financial difficulties, limited physical mobility, loneliness after loss of spouse and close friends, or encountering serious health conditions have been shown to be associated with inappropriate drug use.[15] In the United States (USA), it is estimated that at least one in four older people has a prescription for psychoactive drugs that are open to potential misuse.[33] According to the 2019 National Survey on Drug Use and Health, the frequency of prescription drug misuse in the last year for those aged 50 years and older is given in **Fig. 1**.[34] Common sleep disorders (insomnia) and mental problems in older patients play an important role in prescribing sedative and anxiolytic prescriptions for these cases.[35] In particular, benzodiazepines and opioid analgesics are prescribed for a long time, thus increasing the frequency of side effects associated with these drugs. For example, it has been reported that long-term use of benzodiazepines increases the risk of falls, hip fractures, and traffic accidents, as well as increases the risk of addiction.[36]

Prescription or over-the-counter drug abuse requires attention because of the potential negative consequences. Using drugs that reduce respiratory rate such as central nervous system depressants and opioids, antihistamines, and general anesthetics, especially alcohol, psychotropic, and narcotics, deepens respiratory depression. The increase in prescription drug abuse and misuse increases emergency room visits, overdose deaths, drug use disorders, and treatment applications for addiction.[37]

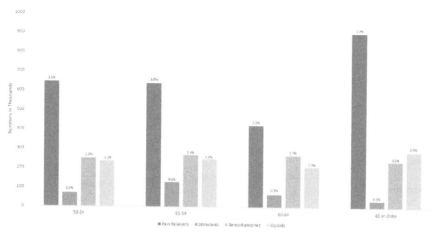

Fig. 1. Misuse of prescribed drugs in past year 2019. (*Data from* Center for Behavioral Health Statistics and Quality. (2020). Results from the 2019 National Survey on Drug Use and Health: Detailed tables. Rockville, MD: Substance Abuse and Mental Health Services Administration. Retrieved from https://www.samhsa.gov/data/.)

Substance-Related Disorder title has been changed as Substance-Related and Addictive Disorders in the Diagnostic and Statistical Manual 5th edition (DSM-5) criteria. Combining abuse and dependence criteria decreases confusion over diagnosis and leads to approach the issue in a broader context. The new 11-item diagnostic criteria are easy to implement in clinical settings yielding early identification and treatment of drug or alcohol problems. DSM-5 change makes it easier for primary care to be reimbursed by insurance to screen for alcohol and drug problems and conduct short counseling sessions.[38] The criteria are also merged to diagnose disorders related to the use of many drugs and substances. Subtitles are defined as alcohol, caffeine, cannabis, hallucinogen, inhalant, opioid, sedative, hypnotic or anxiolytic, stimulant, tobacco, and other (or unknown) substances-related disorders.[39] The drug groups with the most abused in this regard are summarized in **Table 1**.

Opioids

They are used to reduce pain sensation through opioid receptors on the brain and spinal cord. In addition to their pain-reducing properties, they stimulate reward regions in the brain, causing euphoria, which explains the potential for misuse or abuse of opioids.[40] The opioid-analgesic poisoning mortality rate for adults aged 55 to 64 years rose from 1/100,000 in 1999 to nearly 6-fold to 6.3/100,000 in 2011.[41] Chronic pain is an important risk factor for suicide in the older adults, and opioid abuse rates are high in patients with chronic pain.[42] In the USA, the opioid epidemic was declared a national public health emergency in 2017.[43] State and federal policies have been established to reduce opioid prescription in chronic non-malignant pain. A long-term benefit of opioids in pain and function has not been demonstrated with current evidence, and there are no long-term studies to examine outcomes for chronic pain after at least 1 year.[44]

Opioids cause drowsiness, confusion, nausea, constipation, and respiratory depression. The risk of toxicity increases with misuse or abuse with alcohol and sedatives. In long-term regular use, addiction and tolerance may develop, and abrupt termination of use causes withdrawal symptoms. These symptoms include

Table 1	
Commonly abused or misused prescription drugs	
Opioid analgesics	Hydrocodone
	Oxycodone
	Oxymorphone
	Morphine
	Codeine
	Fentanyl
	Meperidine
	Hydromorphone
Stimulants	Amphetamine
	Methylphenidate
Benzodiazepines	Iprazolam
	Triazolam
	Chlorodiazepoxide
	Diazepam
	Lorazepam
Barbiturates	Pentobarbital
	Phenobarbital
Z-drugs	Zaleplon
	Zolpidem
	Eszopiclone
Antidepressants	Bupropion
	Venlafaxine
Antipsychotics	Quetiapine
Gabapentinoids	Pregabalin
	Gabapentin
Dopaminergic Drugs	Levodopa

Data from National Instute on Drug Abuse.Commonly Used Drugs Charts. https://www.drugabuse. gov/drug-topics/commonly-used-drugs-charts#prescription-stimulants. Accessed in 15th May 2021; and Chiappini S, Guirguis A, Corkery J, Schifano F. Understanding the use of prescription and OTC drugs in obtaining illicit highs and the pharmacist role in preventing abuse. The Pharmaceutical Journal. 2020.

restlessness, muscle and bone pain, insomnia, diarrhea, vomiting, cold flashes, and involuntary leg movements.[45] Various risk factors have been identified for opioid misuse and abuse, including sociodemographic factors, pain- and drug-related factors, genetics and environment, underlying psychopathology, and alcohol and substance use disorders. Women are at risk of misusing opioids due to emotional stressors, whereas men tend to abuse opioids for legal and problematic behavioral issues. Chronic physical conditions such as hypertension, arthritis, and arteriosclerosis have been associated with opioid abuse/addiction.[46] Although opioids can be prescribed for reasons other than pain in older adults, the most important opioid indication in this age group is pain. Studies have reported that the use of opioids for indications other than pain increases the risk of benzodiazepine misuse, suicidal ideations, and any substance use disorder in geriatric cases.[47]

Stimulants

The number of stimulant prescriptions for attention deficit hyperactivity disorder has increased in recent years. Stimulants cause an increase in a person's alertness and energy levels, suppression of appetite, and euphoria. Some people use these medications without medical indications to improve mental performance. However, stimulants may cause anxiety and agitation by increasing blood pressure, heart rate, and body temperature. Although misuse is rarely seen in those aged 50 years, their use in the older population is dangerous due to the cardiovascular problems caused by them.[48]

Sedatives

Benzodiazepines are gamma aminobutyric acid (GABA) receptor agonists that provide sedative and anxiolytic effects, primarily used in the treatment of sleep disorders and anxiety. Benzodiazepines can cause euphoria, as well as reduce anxiety and aid sleep. Therefore, they are drugs that are open to abuse for recreational purposes. Long-term (>4 months) and/or high-dose (>10 mg/day diazepam equivalent) use of benzodiazepines is associated with the development of addiction.[33] Benzodiazepines with long half lives, such as flurazepam, are not recommended for use in older adults because of their association with sedative effects, falls, motor vehicle accidents, and memory problems. Withdrawal symptoms include increased heart rate, trembling of hands, insomnia, nausea, vomiting, and anxiety. Generalized seizures can occur in 20% to 30% of users who are not treated for withdrawal symptoms.[33] Long-term use of sedatives, especially benzodiazepines, is more common in women, perceived poor health, and patients with truly poor physical health.

Z-drugs have a different chemical structure, but they act on the same GABA type A receptors in the brain as benzodiazepines and are thought to have fewer side effects and less risk of addiction than benzodiazepines.[49] Barbiturates are classified as sedatives because of their central nervous system calming and sleep effects. The primary therapeutic indications for them are induction of anesthesia and treatment of epilepsy. Most of those who abuse them have experienced other sedatives as well because addiction to them alone is rare.[50]

Antidepressants

Among antidepressants, the dopaminergic effects and stimulant-like activities of bupropion may explain the potential misuse value. In the literature, the recreational use of it is defined as bupropion abuse, including nasal insufflation of crushed tablets and intravenous injection.[51] Venlafaxine is an antidepressant that is a serotonin–norepinephrine reuptake inhibitor. High doses are taken for amphetamine/ecstasy-like euphoria and dissociative effects such as distorted sense of time and numbness. Overdose deaths associated with tachycardia, seizures, coma, and serotonin syndrome have been reported, and addiction problems have been described after prolonged use.[52]

Antipsychotics

Quetiapine is the most abused second-generation antipsychotic because of its sedative and anxiolytic properties. Although the FDA approved its use for schizophrenia and certain types of bipolar and depressive disorders, off-label use is also common for anxiety, depression, dementia behavioral disorders, sleep disorder, and substance use disorder. Information on the misuse of quetiapine is accumulating in the literature. Emergency room admissions for its abuse were reported to almost double between 2005 and 2011.[53] It has been reported that quetiapine misuse is more common in substance abusers or misusers because of its anxiolytic and sedative effects.[54,55]

Gabapentinoids

Gabapentin and pregabalin are used in the treatment of neuropathic pain, fibromyalgia, restless leg syndrome, and epilepsy. They are prescribed off-label in alcohol/narcotic withdrawal and non-neuropathic pain disorders. Gabapentin binds to the auxiliary alpha-2-delta subunit of a voltage-dependent calcium channel, which decrease inward calcium currents and consequently attenuate central neuronal excitability.[56] Pregabalin has a much higher binding affinity for the $\alpha2$-δsubunit and potency than that of gabapentin. Opioid users frequently abuse pregabalin to achieve the desired psychoactive effect (eg, potentiate heroin/cocaine effects), combat opioid withdrawal symptoms, and reduce physical pain.[57] There are reservations for gabapentinoids such as increasing prescription levels over time, users seeing this molecule as an alternative to illegal substances, and increasing drug-related deaths from various countries.[58]

Dopaminergic Agents

Levodopa is often used as a replacement therapy to control motor symptoms in the treatment of Parkinson disease. During the treatment, an impulse control disorder called dopamine dysregulation syndrome (DDS) may be observed, which may cause misuse of dopaminergic drugs by stimulating the central nervous system structures involved in reward signaling including the mesocortical and mesolimbic system. Intake of dopaminergic drugs in higher doses than necessary to control motor symptoms may result in demand for higher doses to the physician.[59] Patients can also misuse levodopa and dopamine agonists. It is stated that personal depressive symptoms and a family or personal history of drug abuse increase the risk for DDS.[60]

PREVENTION AND TREATMENT OF DRUG ABUSE IN OLDER ADULTS

Cognitive problems and psychomotor disorders associated with the use of benzodiazepines and opioids in older adults are common. Defining substance abuse problems in older ages becomes more difficult as signs of addiction or intoxication may appear similar to depression, anxiety, delirium, or dementia or can be attributed to the effects of aging.[61] It should also be noted that health care professionals are less skeptical of abuse in older patients, and as a result, issues related to drug misuse or abuse may not have been adequately reported in patients. Besides, the lack of diagnostic tools and the indistinct clinical consequences of abuse on elderly patients may cause drug abuse to be overlooked.

It would be helpful for medication management for older adults to always have a chart with information about prescription and nonprescription medications that they can share with their health care providers. Limiting exposure to potentially abusive drugs or choosing safer alternative treatments, if possible, involves limiting dose, duration, or number of prescriptions.[62] The effectiveness and adherence to the treatment should be evaluated at regular intervals by informing the patient and their relatives about the side effects of the treatment and the potential for abuse. It is necessary to integrate misuse and abuse screening with cognitive assessment into routine health care to provide comprehensive evaluation tailored to the needs of older patients with multiple needs. Health care professionals should be aware of possible deviations from prescription drugs, recognize cases of abuse and misuse, and design safe treatment regimens for individuals as much as possible, taking into account the possibility of multiple drug abuse.[63] Prescribing should be made in accordance with guidelines to monitor the benefits and risks of chronic opioid therapy.[44]

The lack of validated tools to assess prescription drug problems in older adults leads to underestimation of the prevalence of such problems. However, it has been reported that various irregularities are attempted by the patients and their relatives in order to reach the drugs, which puts a serious economic burden on the health care system. For this reason, electronic data-based prescription drug monitoring programs have been developed in many countries to monitor controlled substances and to inform doctors and pharmacists about this issue.[64]

Treatments aimed at increasing social support and self-esteem are acceptable interventions to reduce problematic prescription drug use. This approach includes identifying causes of non-compliance, informing patients about the importance of following medication management and dosing instructions, and describing the health and functional consequences of prescription drug abuse. Furthermore, encouraging the participation of family members in the treatment process can be effective in increasing the chance of success.[33] Considering the possibility of more severe addiction and the risks of comorbid conditions associated with detoxification in older adults with substance and drug use problems, it should be kept in mind that a special approach is required for these patients. Clinicians should pay close attention to potential drug–drug and drug–disease interactions in older adults being treated for substance-related disorders.

SUMMARY

Despite the evidence that older adults are particularly vulnerable to the misuse and abuse of drugs, insufficient information is available about the screening, evaluation, diagnosis, and treatment. Awareness of all health care professionals involved in the care and treatment of older patients should be increased regarding the problems of misuse and abuse of drugs.

CLINICS CARE POINTS

- Appropriate prescribing is of particular importance in geriatric practice, and several tools have been developed.
- Prescription drugs, such as sedatives, opioids, gabapentinoids, have the potential to misuse or abuse.
- Awareness of the abuse or misuse of prescription drugs in older patients should be expanded because the situation could be easily overlooked, and there are no universally accepted screening and diagnostic tools.

REFERENCES

1. Montamat SC, Cusack B. Overcoming problems with polypharmacy and drug misuse in the elderly. Clin Geriatr Med 1992;8(1):143–58.
2. Unutmaz GD, Soysal P, Tuven B, et al. Costs of medication in older patients: before and after comprehensive geriatric assessment. Clin Interv Aging 2018; 13:607–13.
3. Maher RL, Hanlon J, Hajjar ER. Clinical consequences of polypharmacy in elderly. Expert Opin Drug Saf 2014;13(1):57–65.
4. Mahlknecht A, Krisch L, Nestler N, et al. Impact of training and structured medication review on medication appropriateness and patient-related outcomes in nursing homes: results from the interventional study InTherAKT. BMC Geriatr 2019;19(1):257.

5. Mair A, Fernandez-Llimos F. Polypharmacy management programmes: the SIM-PATHY Project. Eur J Hosp Pharm 2017;24(1):5–6.

6. Rochon PA, Gurwitz JH. The prescribing cascade revisited. Lancet 2017;389(10081):1778–80.

7. Nahin RL, Pecha M, Welmerink DB, et al. Concomitant use of prescription drugs and dietary supplements in ambulatory elderly people. J Am Geriatr Soc 2009;57(7):1197–205.

8. Baruth JM, Gentry MT, Rummans TA, et al. Polypharmacy in older adults: the role of the multidisciplinary team. Hosp Pract (1995) 2020;48(sup1):56–62.

9. Hajjar ER, Cafiero AC, Hanlon JT. Polypharmacy in elderly patients. Am J Geriatr Pharmacother 2007;5(4):345–51.

10. Ates Bulut E, Soysal P, Isik AT. Frequency and coincidence of geriatric syndromes according to age groups: single-center experience in Turkey between 2013 and 2017. Clin Interv Aging 2018;13:1899–905.

11. Halli-Tierney AD, Scarbrough C, Carroll D. Polypharmacy: evaluating risks and deprescribing. Am Fam Physician 2019;100(1):32–8.

12. American geriatrics society 2019 updated AGS beers Criteria® for potentially inappropriate medication use in older adults. J Am Geriatr Soc 2019;67(4):674–94.

13. Piccoliori G, Mahlknecht A, Sandri M, et al. Epidemiology and associated factors of polypharmacy in older patients in primary care: a northern Italian cross-sectional study. BMC Geriatr 2021;21(1):197.

14. Gurwitz JH, Field TS, Harrold LR, et al. Incidence and preventability of adverse drug events among older persons in the ambulatory setting. JAMA 2003;289(9):1107–16.

15. McLarnon ME, Barrett SP, Monaghan TL, et al. Prescription drug misuse across the lifespan: a developmental perspective. In: Verster JC, Brady K, Galanter M, et al, editors. Drug abuse and addiction in medical Illness: causes, consequences and treatment. New York, NY: Springer New York; 2012. p. 213–30.

16. Cooper JA, Cadogan CA, Patterson SM, et al. Interventions to improve the appropriate use of polypharmacy in older people: a Cochrane systematic review. BMJ Open 2015;5(12):e009235.

17. Rankin A, Cadogan CA, Patterson SM, et al. Interventions to improve the appropriate use of polypharmacy for older people. Cochrane Database Syst Rev 2018;9(9):Cd008165.

18. O'Mahony D, O'Sullivan D, Byrne S, et al. STOPP/START criteria for potentially inappropriate prescribing in older people: version 2. Age Ageing 2015;44(2):213–8.

19. Kuhn-Thiel AM, Weiß C, Wehling M. Consensus validation of the FORTA (Fit fOR the Aged) list: a clinical tool for increasing the appropriateness of pharmacotherapy in the elderly. Drugs Aging 2014;31(2):131–40.

20. Hanlon JT, Schmader KE, Samsa GP, et al. A method for assessing drug therapy appropriateness. J Clin Epidemiol 1992;45(10):1045–51.

21. Wenger NS, Shekelle PG. Assessing care of vulnerable elders: ACOVE project overview. Ann Intern Med 2001;135(8 Pt 2):642–6.

22. Holt S, Schmiedl S, Thürmann PA. Potentially inappropriate medications in the elderly: the PRISCUS list. Dtsch Arztebl Int 2010;107(31–32):543–51.

23. Carnahan RM, Lund BC, Perry PJ, et al. The Anticholinergic Drug Scale as a measure of drug-related anticholinergic burden: associations with serum anticholinergic activity. J Clin Pharmacol 2006;46(12):1481–6.

24. Rudolph JL, Salow MJ, Angelini MC, et al. The anticholinergic risk scale and anticholinergic adverse effects in older persons. Arch Intern Med 2008;168(5): 508–13.

25. Cai X, Campbell N, Khan B, et al. Long-term anticholinergic use and the aging brain. Alzheimers Dement 2013;9(4):377–85.

26. Hilmer SN, Mager DE, Simonsick EM, et al. A drug burden index to define the functional burden of medications in older people. Arch Intern Med 2007;167(8): 781–7.

27. Brombo G, Bianchi L, Maietti E, et al. Association of anticholinergic drug burden with cognitive and functional decline over time in older inpatients: results from the CRIME project. Drugs Aging 2018;35(10):917–24.

28. Ruxton K, Woodman RJ, Mangoni AA. Drugs with anticholinergic effects and cognitive impairment, falls and all-cause mortality in older adults: a systematic review and meta-analysis. Br J Clin Pharmacol 2015;80(2):209–20.

29. Steinman MA, Hanlon JT. Managing medications in clinically complex elders: "There's got to be a happy medium. Jama 2010;304(14):1592–601.

30. Smith SM, Dart RC, Katz NP, et al. Classification and definition of misuse, abuse, and related events in clinical trials: ACTTION systematic review and recommendations. Pain 2013;154(11):2287–96.

31. Cotto JH, Davis E, Dowling GJ, et al. Gender effects on drug use, abuse, and dependence: a special analysis of results from the National Survey on drug use and health. Gend Med 2010;7(5):402–13.

32. Culberson JW, Ziska M. Prescription drug misuse/abuse in the elderly. Geriatrics 2008;63(9):22–31.

33. Simoni-Wastila L, Yang HK. Psychoactive drug abuse in older adults. Am J Geriatr Pharmacother 2006;4(4):380–94.

34. Center for Behavioral Health Statistics and Quality. Results from the 2019 national survey on drug use and health: detailed tables. Rockville, MD: Substance Abuse and Mental Health Services Administration; 2020. Available at: https://www.samhsa.gov/data/.

35. Prinz PN, Vitiello MV, Raskind MA, et al. Geriatrics: sleep disorders and aging. N Engl J Med 1990;323(8):520–6.

36. Griffiths RR, Johnson MW. Relative abuse liability of hypnotic drugs: a conceptual framework and algorithm for differentiating among compounds. J Clin Psychiatry 2005;66(Suppl 9):31–41.

37. Jones CM, McAninch JK. Emergency department visits and overdose deaths from combined use of opioids and benzodiazepines. Am J Prev Med 2015; 49(4):493–501.

38. Hasin DS, O'Brien CP, Auriacombe M, et al. DSM-5 criteria for substance use disorders: recommendations and rationale. Am J Psychiatry 2013;170(8):834–51.

39. Association AP. Diagnostic and statistical manual of mental disorders. Washington, DC: American Psychiatric Association; 2013.

40. Pergolizzi J, Böger RH, Budd K, et al. Opioids and the management of chronic severe pain in the elderly: consensus statement of an International expert panel with focus on the six clinically most often used World Health Organization Step III opioids (buprenorphine, fentanyl, hydromorphone, methadone, morphine, oxycodone). Pain Pract 2008;8(4):287–313.

41. Chen LH, Hedegaard H, Warner M. Drug-poisoning deaths involving opioid analgesics: United States, 1999-2011. NCHS Data Brief 2014;(166):1–8.

42. Webster LR. Risk factors for opioid-use disorder and overdose. Anesth Analg 2017;125(5):1741–8.

43. U.S. Department of health and Human Services. U.S acting secretary declares public health emergency to address national opioid crisis 2017. Available at: https://www.hhs.gov/about/news/2017/10/26/hhs-acting-secretary-declares-public-health-emergency-address-national-opioid-crisis.html.

44. Dowell D, Haegerich TM, Chou R. CDC guideline for prescribing opioids for chronic pain–United States, 2016. JAMA 2016;315(15):1624–45.

45. Jones CM, Lurie PG, Throckmorton DC. Effect of US drug enforcement administration's rescheduling of hydrocodone combination analgesic products on opioid analgesic prescribing. JAMA Intern Med 2016;176(3):399–402.

46. Kaye AD, Jones MR, Kaye AM, et al. Prescription opioid abuse in chronic pain: an updated review of opioid abuse predictors and strategies to curb opioid abuse: Part 1. Pain Physician 2017;20(2s):S93–109.

47. Schepis TS, Wastila L, Ammerman B, et al. Prescription opioid misuse Motives in US older adults. Pain Med 2020;21(10):2237–43.

48. Spiller HA, Hays HL, Aleguas A Jr. Overdose of drugs for attention-deficit hyperactivity disorder: clinical presentation, mechanisms of toxicity, and management. CNS drugs 2013;27(7):531–43.

49. Badrakalimuthu VR, Rumball D, Wagle A. Drug misuse in older people: old problems and new challenges. Adv Psychiatr Treat 2010;16(6):421–9.

50. Weaver MF. Prescription sedative misuse and abuse. Yale J Biol Med 2015;88(3):247–56.

51. Stall N, Godwin J, Juurlink D. Bupropion abuse and overdose. CMAJ 2014;186(13):1015.

52. Leonard JB, Klein-Schwartz W. Characterization of intentional-abuse venlafaxine exposures reported to poison control centers in the United States. Am J Drug Alcohol Abuse 2019;45(4):421–6.

53. Mattson ME, Albright VA, Yoon J, et al. Emergency department visits involving misuse and abuse of the antipsychotic quetiapine: results from the drug abuse warning network (DAWN). Subst Abuse 2015;9:39–46.

54. McLarnon ME, Fulton HG, MacIsaac C, et al. Characteristics of quetiapine misuse among clients of a community-based methadone maintenance program. J Clin Psychopharmacol 2012;32(5):721–3.

55. Cubała WJ, Springer J. Quetiapine abuse and dependence in psychiatric patients: a systematic review of 25 case reports in the literature. J Substance Use 2014;19(5):388–93.

56. van Hooft JA, Dougherty JJ, Endeman D, et al. Gabapentin inhibits presynaptic Ca(2+) influx and synaptic transmission in rat hippocampus and neocortex. Eur J Pharmacol 2002;449(3):221–8.

57. Buttram ME, Kurtz SP. Descriptions of gabapentin misuse and associated behaviors among a sample of opioid (Mis)users in south Florida. J Psychoactive Drugs 2021;53(1):47–54.

58. Schifano F. Misuse and abuse of pregabalin and gabapentin: cause for concern? CNS Drugs 2014;28(6):491–6.

59. Giovannoni G, O'Sullivan JD, Turner K, et al. Hedonistic homeostatic dysregulation in patients with Parkinson's disease on dopamine replacement therapies. J Neurol Neurosurg Psychiatry 2000;68(4):423–8.

60. Cilia R, Siri C, Canesi M, et al. Dopamine dysregulation syndrome in Parkinson's disease: from clinical and neuropsychological characterisation to management and long-term outcome. J Neurol Neurosurg Psychiatry 2014;85(3):311–8.

61. Maree RD, Marcum ZA, Saghafi E, et al. A systematic review of opioid and benzodiazepine misuse in older adults. Am J Geriatr Psychiatry 2016;24(11): 949–63.
62. Paulozzi LJ, Kilbourne EM, Shah NG, et al. A history of being prescribed controlled substances and risk of drug overdose death. Pain Med 2012;13(1): 87–95.
63. Riggs P. Non-medical use and abuse of commonly prescribed medications. Curr Med Res Opin 2008;24(3):869–77.
64. Kirschner N, Ginsburg J, Sulmasy LS. Prescription drug abuse: executive summary of a policy position paper from the American College of Physicians. Ann Intern Med 2014;160(3):198–200.

Over-The-Counter Remedies in Older Adults

Patterns of Use, Potential Pitfalls, and Proposed Solutions

Delavar Safari, BA*, Elisabeth C. DeMarco, BS, Lillian Scanlon, BS,
George T. Grossberg, MD

KEYWORDS

- Adverse effects • Drug–drug interactions • FDA regulations
- Nonprescription/OTC medications • Dietary supplements
- Geriatric/older adult population

KEY POINTS

- Prevalence of OTC medication, supplement, vitamin, and herbal remedy use among the older population is high both in the United States and globally.
- The older population is at increased risk of inappropriate OTC product use and medication errors which can result in drug–drug interactions, drug–disease interactions, and adverse drug reactions.
- The FDA provides national standards for many OTC products but dietary supplements, including herbal remedies, vitamins, minerals, and amino acids are not bound by these standards and are not subject to FDA pre-approval. International standards are lacking.
- Accessible educational information to promote informed decision-making and improved healthcare provider–patient communication is needed to better protect the older population.

INTRODUCTION

Millions of Americans extensively use over-the-counter (OTC) products as an accessible and effective solution to self-medicate commonly occurring conditions[1] and the number of available OTC medications is rapidly increasing, with more than 300,000 OTC drug products available today.[2] According to the Consumer Healthcare Products Association, Americans take OTC medications most commonly for upper respiratory grievances; pain management; heartburn; constipation; and oral, skin, and eye care.[3]

While OTC medications can be obtained without a healthcare practitioner's authorization because they are generally considered to be safe for the general population,

Department of Psychiatry & Behavioral Neuroscience, Division of Geriatric Psychiatry, School of Medicine, Saint Louis University, 1438 S Grand Boulevard, St Louis, MO 63104, USA
* Corresponding author.
E-mail address: delavar.safari@health.slu.edu

Clin Geriatr Med 38 (2022) 99–118
https://doi.org/10.1016/j.cger.2021.07.005
0749-0690/22/© 2021 Elsevier Inc. All rights reserved.
geriatric.theclinics.com

several safety issues and adverse effects can arise. The older adult population is at elevated risk as many commonly purchased OTC products contain ingredients deemed to be potentially inappropriate for this population.[4] For example, diphenhydramine, included in numerous OTC products marketed for various symptoms (for allergies, cough and cold, and as sleep aids), can impair cognition, cause dizziness, and may increase the risk of fall.[5] OTC analgesics such as ibuprofen may cause bleeding and ulcers, increase blood pressure, reduce the effectiveness of antihypertensive medications, and cause kidney damage in patients with congestive heart failure and renal disease.[6,7] Despite recent advances in monitoring and documenting potential medication risks in the older adult population,[8–10] age-related changes in pharmacokinetics and pharmacodynamics are still not well understood.

In addition, older adults more often suffer from multimorbidity, the co-occurrence of two or more diseases, increasing the likelihood of polypharmacy. This may not only lead to an increased risk of inappropriate drug use and medication errors but also result in drug–drug interactions, drug–disease interactions, and adverse drug reactions.[11] These risks may not be intuitive to the patient, and appropriate use of OTC products can be better assessed with a healthcare provider's expertise. Here, we review the use of OTC medications among older adults. We summarize possible, notable adverse effects of OTC products; examine current regulations; and propose solutions for current challenges around OTC product misuse for providers, patients, and regulators.

EPIDEMIOLOGY

OTC product use among older adults is widespread in the United States (U.S.) and internationally. Approximately 40% of community-dwelling older adults aged 62 to 85 years report use of OTC medications, and more than 60% report the use of dietary supplements.[12] Older adults frequently manage pain with nonprescription acetaminophen and the nonsteroidal anti-inflammatory drugs (NSAIDs) ibuprofen and aspirin.[13] Recent studies suggest NSAIDs are used by up to 47.6% of older adults[14] and inappropriate use of NSAIDs may occur in 13% to 72% of older adult NSAID users.[14,15] Among residents of residential aged care facilities, 23.3% used at least one NSAID, and 14.8% used an NSAID long term.[16]

Anticholinergic drugs, laxatives, complementary and alternative medicines (CAMs), including herbal products, and dietary supplements like vitamins are also commonly used.[3,17] Common anticholinergic drugs include first-generation antihistamines such as diphenhydramine, doxylamine, and dimenhydrinate. These can be found in products including Benadryl, nighttime or "PM" products, and medications used to treat allergies, insomnia, cold and cough, motion sickness, and other acute or chronic conditions.[18–20] Among older adults, as many as 15.3% to 19.3% report dissatisfactions with sleep duration and quality.[21,22] Among older adults reporting insomnia, 18% to 38.6% used an OTC sleep aid.[18,22,23] While adults from different age groups demonstrate similar prevalence in the use of OTC sleep aids, many adults aged older than 65 years (37% of people aged 65%–74%, and 47% of people aged 75+) used the medications over the recommended 14 days compared with adults aged younger than 64 years (21%).[18] This is concerning because product labeling for diphenhydramine and doxylamine advises patients to stop use and consult a healthcare provider if sleeplessness persists for more than 2 weeks, and both products are considered potentially inappropriate for use by older adults.[24]

Constipation is also common among older adults.[25] While prevalence estimates vary, approximately 33.5% of people aged 60 to 101 years suffer from constipation, with women and nursing home residents being more often affected.[26–29] While reports of the extent of laxative use in the U.S. vary widely from 3% to 59% in the general population,[30] and the laxative use is suggested high in older adults due to increased prevalence of constipation, conclusive studies are missing, especially for the prevalence of OTC laxative use among older adults. One study of South Australian adults aged older than 65 years indicates laxatives are second only to analgesics as the most commonly used OTC medication.[31] Furthermore, 17% of older patients admitted to the cardiology service in a tertiary care medical center in the U.S. reported OTC laxative use,[32] whereas 41.5% of older adults with disabilities reported laxative use, primarily for chronic constipation.[33]

Beyond nonprescription medications, the use of dietary supplements (including vitamins, herbals, and minerals) has increased from nearly 50% in 2005 to 2006 to more than 60% in 2010 to 2011[12] and older adults more often report the use of dietary supplements compared with younger adults.[34] Up to 70% of older adults in the U.S. reported using more than one dietary supplement in the past 30 days and 29% reported taking more than four products.[35] Improving and maintaining overall health and prophylaxis are by far the most common reasons given for the use of dietary supplements.[35,36] Older adults use dietary supplements more often for specific reasons such as heart health, lower cholesterol, and healthy joints and bones compared with younger adults.[34] The most frequently reported products were multivitamin or mineral (39%), vitamin D only (26%), and omega-3 fatty acids (22%).[35] In addition, intake of herbal products such as spearmint, chamomile, aloe vera, and garlic has increased steadily from 3% in 1990[37] to 12% in 1997[38] to around 50% in 2003[39] and 2011[40] and falling slightly to around 40% in 2015.[41] Interestingly, baby boomers (born between 1945 and 1969) were more likely than pre-boomers (born before 1945) to report using CAMs in a study using data from 2001 to 2003.[42] While multivitamin use was comparable among age groups, more than double the number of baby boomers used herbal treatments compared with pre-boomers in this study (16.9% to 7.3%, respectively).[42] Given this trend, future generations of older adults might be even more likely to use CAMs. Several demographic factors have consistently been found to be associated with vitamin/mineral supplement use: White race, female gender, increased education, and higher socioeconomic status.[43]

ADVERSE EFFECTS OF COMMON OVER-THE-COUNTER PRODUCTS IN OLDER ADULTS

While OTC medications are generally thought to be safe to use, 41% of the general public believes nonprescription medications are too weak to cause any problems.[44] The perception of low risks associated with OTC products is more pronounced in older adults.[45] In reality, a growing body of research suggests elevated risks of adverse effects for the older population. As a recent study suggests, these are often caused by unintentional misuse of OTC products in combination with prescription drugs.[46] Here, we present a selection of commonly observed adverse effects that healthcare providers should be aware of and communicate to their older adult patients.

Side Effects of Common over-the-Counter Drugs, Herbs, and Supplements

Side effects are usually regarded as an undesirable secondary effect that occurs in addition to the desired therapeutic effect and can be dependent on age, weight, gender, ethnicity, and general health. Serious side effects of OTC medications (**Table 1**) and supplements (**Table 2**) particularly occur in the older adult population due to changes in pharmacokinetic properties. While the absorption of a drug is not

Table 1 Common OTC drugs and associated adverse effects	
Drug	**Major adverse effects**
Acetaminophen	Hepatotoxicity[47]; Acute liver failure[47]
NSAIDs	Gastrointestinal toxicity (dyspepsia, peptic ulcer disease, bleeding)[48]; Acute kidney injury, hypertension, electrolyte disturbances[49–51]; cardiovascular events (myocardial infarction, stroke)[52]; neurologic effects[53] (rare)
Antihistamines	Anticholinergic effects (blurred vision, xerostomia, urinary retention, tachycardia, nausea, constipation, agitation, confusion, cognitive dysfunction, delirium)[54]
Laxatives	Abdominal pain, constipation, diarrhea, increased thirst, abdominal distention, anorectal pain, nausea, malaise[55–57]

affected by aging due to passive absorption, the elimination halftime can be changed due to age-related increases in body fat, decreases in total body water, and reduction in plasma proteins.[58–60] Common examples include:

Acetaminophen

Acetaminophen, one of the most widely used OTC drugs in the older adult population, is recommended by the American Geriatrics Society (AGS) as the first-line agent for mild-to-moderate chronic pain in older adults due to its favorable safety profile.[48] However, it can cause acute hepatotoxicity at high doses through the formation of the toxic metabolite, N-acetyl-p-benzoquinone imine (NAPQI).[47] NAPQI under normal conditions is suggested to conjugate with glutathione and then be eliminated through renal excretion. In overdosed patients, however, massive NAPQI formation can cause glutathione depletion and binding to cellular proteins resulting in severe hepatocellular injury.[61] This can be exacerbated in older adults as there is considerable evidence that glutathione tissue levels tend to decline with age.[62,63] Acetaminophen toxicity is responsible for 46% of acute liver failure cases in the U.S.[47]

Nonsteroidal anti-inflammatory drugs (NSAIDs) are another popular class of analgesics and are generally considered second-line for pain treatment if acetaminophen fails to control pain effectively or when treating an inflammatory type of pain where acetaminophen has limited efficacy.[64] The AGS recommends NSAIDs use for only short periods during episodic flares because extended use can result in gastrointestinal toxicity including dyspepsia, peptic ulcer disease, and bleeding.[48] Cyclooxygenase (COX) is an enzyme involved in the synthesis of prostaglandins, which protect the mucosal lining of the GI tract. Many NSAIDs block the COX-1 and COX-2 enzymes, which impairs prostaglandin synthesis and results in injury.[65] This is especially critical in the older population as age greater than 65 years, prior dyspepsia, and previous upper GI injury (ulcer, bleeding, perforation) increase the risk of NSAID-associated GI events.[66] NSAIDs are also linked to an increase in cardiovascular events, such as myocardial infarction and stroke, both of which are more often associated with increased age[67] and potentially due to reduced production of prostaglandin I2 by the vascular endothelium, which could predispose to injury.[52] While renal side effects of NSAIDs are less common compared with GI and cardiovascular risks, NSAIDs-dependent COX inhibition with subsequent reduction in prostaglandin synthesis can lead to renal vasoconstriction and consequently reduced renal perfusion and aberrant renal function.[49] Various forms of renal failures have been described, including acute deterioration of renal function, renal papillary

Table 2
Common herbs and supplements and associated adverse effects or drug interactions

Herb/supplement	Major adverse effects
Calcium and Vitamin D	Nephrolithiasis; Constipation, Hypercalcemia; Hypercalciuria[82,83]
Green tea extract (*Camellia sinensis L.*)	Hepatotoxicity[84]
Ginkgo biloba	Case reports of bleeding risk[85] and conflicting evidence of altered warfarin metabolism, with subsequent increased bleeding risk[86–90]
Aloe vera, cranberry, flaxseed, garlic	No serious adverse events[91]
Ginseng	May induce CYP3A activity[92]
St. John's wort	May reduce effectiveness of warfarin, digoxin, and other prescription medications[93,94] Cases of serotonin syndrome reported when taken together with SSRIs[95]
Vitamin E	Use correlated with increased risk of bleeding in patients being treated with warfarin[96]

necrosis, acute interstitial nephritis, hyperkalemia, and sodium, and fluid retention.[49–51] Risk of chronic kidney disease progression in older adults is associated with high cumulative NSAIDs exposure.[68] This is concerning as a study showed around 15% of individuals living in residential aged care facilities used an NSAID regularly.[16] Neurologic effects are rare with NSAIDs; however, older adults who take indomethacin may be at a higher risk for confusion and psychosis,[53] thus indomethacin should be used with caution.[53]

Antihistamines

Antihistamines, such as diphenhydramine, hydroxyzine, doxylamine, and dimenhydrinate, are known to cause anticholinergic side effects, to which the geriatric population is particularly susceptible.[24] These adverse effects include blurred vision, xerostomia, urinary retention, tachycardia, nausea, constipation, agitation, confusion, cognitive disfunction, and delirium.[54] For diphenhydramine, the most commonly used OTC first-generation antihistamine, cognitive effects are of special concern, as grogginess, drowsiness, and confusion, reduced alertness, diminished memory task performance, and impaired episodic memory have been associated with diphenhydramine.[69–72] In hospitalized older adults, this can result in increased length of hospital stay.[73] Generally, drugs with anticholinergic side effects are inappropriate for use in older adults based on the updated Beer's criteria.[24]

Laxatives

Laxatives are also frequently used by the older adult population and include bulk-forming agents, osmotic and stimulant laxatives, and others.[74] Bulk-forming agents increase the water absorbency capacity of stool leading to improved stool frequency and consistency[75] but may cause abdominal cramping or bloating.[76] Polyethylene glycol, an osmotic laxative, usually causes minimal adverse effects when consumed as recommended.[76,77] When administered in high doses, however, it may cause nausea, abdominal bloating, cramping, and flatulence and can result in excessive stool frequency, especially in older nursing home residents.[55–57]

Healthcare providers are often not involved in laxative product selection and an average of three laxative products are used before consulting a healthcare professional.[78] This is especially critical in older adults as abdominal discomfort, electrolyte imbalance, allergic reactions, and impaired kidney function have been reported with laxative use.[79–81] Additionally, cases of severe hypermagnesemia have been reported when magnesium-based laxatives were used in patients with renal disease.[79]

Herbs and supplements

Adverse effects have also been noted with the use of herbs and supplements (**Table 2**), particularly when taken above the recommended dietary allowance. For example, calcium and vitamin D supplementation is commonly used for the prevention of osteoporosis, a disease common in older adults, but may lead to nephrolithiasis, constipation, hypercalcemia, and hypercalciuria when taken in excess.[82,83] Examples of Commonly Consumed Herbal Supplements Include

Green tea extract

Green tea extract (*Camellia sinensis L.*) has been marketed as an antioxidant, a weight management strategy, and to lower the risk of cancer but has been associated with hepatotoxicity.[84] Epigallocatechin-3-gallate (EGCG), a catechin in green tea induces reactive oxygen species that may be involved in hepatocellular injury.[84]

Gingko biloba

Ginkgo biloba has been touted to be effective in the treatment of anxiety, cognitive decline, glaucoma, and other diseases,[97] yet there have been case reports of bleeding, including subdural hematoma and subarachnoid hemorrhage.[85] It has been suggested that ginkgo biloba may also prolong bleeding times in patients already on prescription blood thinners, such as warfarin.[86,87] However, randomized controlled trials designed to detect side effects from ginkgo found no interactions with warfarin[88] or any effect on bleeding time, coagulation parameters, or platelet activity.[89,90,98] The conflicting data regarding a causal association between bleeding events and concomitant ginkgo and warfarin use call for further studies.

A systematic review of herbal medication effectiveness and possible adverse events concluded herbals were generally better tolerated than synthetic medications.[91] Supplements such as aloe vera, cranberry, flaxseed, garlic, and ginseng were not found to be associated with any serious adverse events.[91] The body of knowledge surrounding adverse effects of herbs and supplements is continuing to evolve, especially their tolerability and side effects in older adults.

Interactions of OTC Drugs, Herbs, and Supplements with Prescription Drugs

Drug–drug interactions may result from pharmacokinetic interactions (ie, alterations in drug absorption, volume of distribution, metabolism, or excretion), pharmacodynamic interactions (ie, additive, synergistic, or antagonistic effects that occur despite unaltered plasma levels of the drugs), pharmaceutical incompatibility, a combination of these mechanisms, or other unknown mechanisms.[99] While there is no consensus definition of what constitutes polypharmacy, approximately 30% of adults aged older than 65 years in developed countries take five or more medications.[100] These numbers are even higher in long-term care settings and the context of end-of-life care.[101,102] In addition, the prevalence of general vitamin and mineral supplement use can be up to 85%.[17] Polypharmacy increases the risk of drug–drug interactions, especially if OTC products are used in combination with prescription drugs. The prevalence of inappropriate medication use in older adult populations ranges from 11.5% to 62.5%.[103]

Both Acetaminophen and NSAIDs interact with numerous prescription drugs and alcohol. Acetaminophen may enhance the hepatotoxic effects of alcohol and dasatinib and sorafenib, two kinase inhibitors.[104] Probenecid has been shown to reduce the clearance of acetaminophen, increasing the risk of toxicity.[105] Acetaminophen also interacts with barbiturates,[106] carbamazepine,[107] phenytoin,[106] imatinib,[108] lamotrigine,[109] metyrapone,[110] phenylephrine,[111] rifampin,[112] warfarin,[113] and others. Close monitoring is recommended when administering acetaminophen with any of these drugs, but there are few absolute contraindications.[114] NSAIDs may cause gastrointestinal bleeding or increased blood pressure in older adults when used concomitantly with other medications. Some affected drugs include antiplatelets, angiotensin-converting-enzyme inhibitors, corticosteroids, diuretics, methotrexate, Selective serotonin reuptake inhibitors (SSRI), and anticoagulants.[51] Diphenhydramine and other antihistamines should be avoided in combination with other central nervous system (CNS) depressants, as the effect may be enhanced.[115]

Herbs and supplements can also interact with other drugs. One of the first herb-drug interactions discovered was St. John's wort, a flower used for its possible antidepressant effects and a potent inducer of the cytochrome P-450 enzymes and intestinal P-glycoprotein.[116] Concomitant use of St. John's wort can reduce the effectiveness of warfarin, digoxin, and many other prescription medications.[93,94] In the older adult population, cases of serotonin syndrome have been reported when St. John's wort was taken together with SSRIs.[95] Limited evidence suggests ginseng may induce CYP3A activity and close monitoring of any patients taking ginseng along with CYP3A substrates, such as midazolam, cyclosporine, or tacrolimus, is recommended to ensure a therapeutic response.[92] Vitamin E, common in many multivitamins taken by older adults, has been linked to increased risk of bleeding in patients being treated with warfarin.[96]

Food–Drug Interactions

In addition to OTC drugs and herbs, interactions between foods and prescription drugs have also been found, such as the inhibitory effect of grapefruit juice on the CYP3A4 isoenzyme.[117] The resulting increased bioavailability of certain calcium channel blockers and HMG-CoA reductase inhibitors can result in adverse events such as hypotension.[117] Warfarin efficacy can be decreased by consumption of vitamin K-rich, green, leafy vegetables, which increases the risk of clot formation.[118] Consumption of dairy products can significantly decrease absorption of fluoroquinolone and tetracycline antibiotics due to the formation of cation complexes.[119] Patients taking MAO inhibitors, rarely used for treatment-resistant depression, can develop a hypertensive crisis following the consumption of tyramine-rich foods such as red wine, chocolate, meat, and cheese. Tyramine is an indirect sympathomimetic amine and acts as a vasopressor.[120] Healthcare providers should screen for possible dietary causes of these adverse effects.

REGULATORY OVERSIGHT OF OVER-THE-COUNTER PRODUCTS IN THE U.S. AND GLOBALLY
Food and Drug Administration Oversight

Widespread use of OTC pharmaceuticals, herbal remedies, and dietary supplements and the significant potential for adverse effects creates a unique regulatory opportunity to monitor product quality, safety, and efficacy. There are two regulatory pathways for OTC drugs.[121] The OTC Drug Review evaluates the safety and effectiveness of OTC drug products already on the market issuing drug monographs which specify active ingredients, uses (indications), doses, labeling, and testing under which an OTC drug is generally recognized as safe and effective.[122] New OTC drugs within the same category can be manufactured to these standards and marketed without FDA pre-approval.[121,122] OTC drugs that do not conform with an existing category must be reviewed by the NDA process.[123]

In contrast to an OTC drug, dietary supplements are regulated by the FDA via the 1994 Dietary Supplement Health and Education Act (DSHEA).[124] While pre-marketing approval of dietary supplements is not required,[124] manufacturers are expected to provide evidence to demonstrate the reasonable expectation of their product's safety for example, through Good Manufacturing Practices (GMP).[124,125] However, private implementation of these practices does not establish legally enforceable responsibilities and often leads to a lack of uniformity.[125] While DSHEA provides the FDA with regulatory authority to protect consumers from adulterated dietary supplements,[124] the FDA bears the burden of proof to deem a dietary supplement adulterated.[124,126] To continuously monitor substances currently available, the FDA conducts adverse event reporting by physicians, consumers, and patients via MedWatch.[127]

Medical foods are defined by the FDA as substances used for dietary management of a disease or health condition that requires special nutrient needs beyond modification of a normal diet and are administered under the supervision of a physician.[105,128,129] As with dietary supplements, medical foods are not subject to pre-market approval, must comply with GMP and registration provisions, and must adhere to truthful advertising claims.[128,129] Medical foods are regulated as foods by the FDA unless a specific health claim is made that implies treatment, prevention, relief, or diagnosis of a specific disease.[128] This regulatory strategy leaves a substantial gray area as food and nutrition are increasingly incorporated as part of health management, especially in the older population.[130,131]

Advertising and promotion of both food and dietary supplements are regulated by the Federal Trade Commission (FTC) and the advertiser is responsible for ensuring the accuracy of implicit and explicit claims and bears the responsibility for substantiating all claims.[132] Health claims made by foods must meet several general standards established by the FDA (**Box 1**).[133]

Box 1
General standards for health claims established by FDA and FTC

General Standards Include but are not Limited to:

- Authorizing only categories of claims where the diet–disease relationship is supported by "significant scientific evidence"

- Establishing maximum limits for total fat, saturated fat, cholesterol, and sodium, such that foods in excess of these limits cannot bear any health claims

- Defining a threshold amount (minimum or maximum) for the amount of the substance which is the subject of the health claim

- Requiring some minimal nutritional value for any food to bear a health claim

- Requiring the identification of factors which affect the diet–disease relationship, outside dietary intake of that substance

Data from Commission FT. Enforcement Policy Statement on Food Advertising. In: Commission FT, ed 1994. https://www.ftc.gov/public-statements/1994/05/enforcement-policy-statement-food-advertising

United States Pharmacopeia Approval

The United States Pharmacopeia (USP) Convention is a non-profit organization founded in 1906 and develops standards for pharmaceutical products with the FDA.[134] The USP National Formulary, first created in 1938, contains standards for pharmaceuticals and many dietary supplements.[126,134,135] In addition, USP offers third-party verification services to manufacturers[136] and maintains a database of all verified products with monographs available worldwide.[134,137]

Global Standards for OTC Products

Increasing globalization of markets, supply chains, and manufacturing introduces greater challenges for the regulation of OTC products. International standards for regulation and scrutiny of OTC products vary widely across countries and classes of products. These challenges are exemplified when considering products purchased from international websites which may not be subject to regulatory controls of the country where the purchaser resides.[138] Furthermore, terminology and classification vary widely, such that the same substance might be considered a supplement in the EU and a medicine in Canada. International efforts are underway to improve global standards.[139,140]

PROPOSED SOLUTIONS
Accessible Educational Information to Promote Informed Decisions

We still know surprisingly little about the ways older adults select OTC medications, decide when to start or stop using, actually use these medications, or involve clinicians and family members in these decisions.[141] One study used interview findings, in-store shopping observations, and laboratory-based simulated shopping findings to build a model that distinguishes between two decision-making pathways, a habit-based and a deliberation-based process.[19] This model can be used to design directions for consumer interventions related to OTC medication use and safety. For example, interventions targeting habit-based decision-making could support safer habits for older adults, that is, by replacing an existing routine with another. Deliberation-based decisions could be supported with education, product labeling, or decision aids using personalized, just-in-time information.

In fact, most overdoses in older adults are unintentional and may result from dementia, improper use, or mistaken identities.[142] Better education about possible risks for the patient is highly recommended. The FDA provides valuable resources for consumers online.[143]

Furthermore, patients who cannot understand the label on an OTC product cannot truly make an informed decision. According to the most recent report of Health Literacy in the U.S., adults aged 65 years and older tend to have lower health literacy levels than adults younger than 65 years.[144] While the FDA has implemented guidelines to improve labeling including the establishment of a consistent order of listing information and using "easy-to-understand" language,[145] multiple studies call for improved labeling.[146,147] For an older patient to read the label about potential adverse events, cognitive functions, including memory, concentration, word recognition, and adequate vision, must be intact. Any deficit in one of these areas will affect the comprehension and interpretation of risks associated with medication.[146] Graphical displays have been shown to lead to more accurate interpretations of risks by older adults[148,149] and may therefore be worth considering.

The pharmacist can also play a role in educating consumers. Studies showed that consumers provided with an ask-the-pharmacist service demonstrated a high rate of questions for pharmacists regarding effectiveness and safety.[150] However, other studies indicate consumers do not seek out advice if the pharmacist is not perceived as available, approachable, or accessible.[19] Health information technology (HIT) is a promising approach for addressing the challenges of communicating health information.[141,151] HIT focuses on the use of technology to assist consumers, practitioners, and other stakeholders with health-related tasks. However, the effectiveness of HIT often depends on the usability of the technology, which is especially critical for older adults. Several studies are currently developing and reviewing new tools, especially for older adults.[152]

Better Healthcare Provider–Patient Communication

According to estimates, only about 37% to 50% of healthcare providers ask about their patients' OTC drug use and only 50% of patients reported their OTC use to healthcare providers.[153–156] Inadequate communication of OTC product use may result in ineffective disease management or unrecognized, potentially harmful drug-herb/drug-supplement interactions. It is therefore highly recommended for healthcare professionals to inquire about OTC use in their patients. Clinicians must ask questions that will elicit, address, and, if possible, change patients' misperceptions of OTC medications. One productive approach is to recognize the commonsense rationale for the therapy, address concerns about potential adverse effects, and make the regimen as convenient and easy to follow as possible.[157] To that end, continuing education for physicians is crucial. The NIH provides a plethora of helpful information online such as free video lectures, a list of recent literature reviews, and evidence reports.[158,159] While there is little research about the effectiveness of health care professional (HCP) educational tools, focused medical education can improve HCP knowledge and attitudes toward disease management.[160] Furthermore, OTC products receive little attention in medical school curricula. A pilot study evaluating student attitudes and knowledge in connection with a new curriculum incorporating teachings about OTC medications in a longitudinal family medicine clerkship showed medical students found teaching about OTC medications to be useful and students demonstrated significant improvement on a fund of knowledge test.[161] Additionally, encouraging patients and providers alike to use the USP registry of approved products[137] can increase confidence in the quality of OTC products.

Updated Regulations

Policy governing the approval, quality, and monitoring of OTC products is another avenue to improve patient safety. This could include instituting a national supplement registry overseen by the FDA or another appropriate entity, or requiring companies to submit product names, ingredients, and contact information before entering the market.[162] Expanding on the existing NIH Dietary Supplement Label Database[163] and NIH Dietary Supplement Ingredient Database[164] would be one way to approach a national registry. These projects are currently intended for research applications and information is supplied by several collaborating organizations.[163,164] Such a registry could be regularly screened for illegal ingredients such as registered pharmaceutical products, triggering immediate warnings and preventing products from entering the market. While continued updates to the USP monographs would standardize manufacturer's quality control efforts, mandating the use of these standards or other publicly available pharmacopeia standards for quality and GMP would further protect the American public.[126] Regulating dietary supplements as pharmaceuticals rather than foods would align quality and manufacturing standards for dietary supplements with those of OTC drug products.[126] Short of this, designating an official compendium for food standards would allow laws surrounding adulteration to be applied to dietary supplements, which are currently classified as foods.[165] Increasing the safety of the consumer through proactive monitoring and regulation of OTC products can be accomplished with many policy solutions.

SUMMARY

The prevalence of OTC medication, supplement, vitamin, and herbal remedy use among older adults is high both in the U.S. and globally. While OTC products provide an important tool for self-medication, the older population is at increased risk of inappropriate OTC product use and medication errors which can result in drug-drug interactions, drug–disease interactions, and adverse drug reactions. The FDA provides national standards for OTC generic drugs, but dietary supplements, including herbal remedies, vitamins, minerals, and amino acids are not subject to FDA pre-approval. International standards are lacking. Few older patients choose to inform their healthcare provider about the OTC products they take, and healthcare providers often fail to inquire about the patient's OTC use. Accessible educational information to promote informed decision-making, updated national and international regulations, and improved healthcare provider–patient communication are needed to better protect the older population from misuse of OTC products.

FUNDING SOURCES

The authors have no funding sources to disclose.

CLINICS CARE POINTS

- Prevalence of OTC medication, supplement, vitamin, and herbal remedy use among the elderly is high in the United States.
- The older population is at increased risk of inappropriate OTC product use. Certain products should be avoided (NSAIDs, drugs with anticholinergic side effects and members of the Beer's list).
- Adverse effects are less well understood in older adults therefore careful monitoring is needed.
- As many patients do not disclose OTC use, health care providers should inquire about OTC use of the patient.
- Accessible educational information for healthcare providers and patients is needed and improved healthcare provider - patient communication is necessary.
- While the FDA provides national standards for many OTC products, dietary supplements, including herbal remedies, vitamins, minerals, and amino acids are not bound by these standards. This calls for changes in regulatory oversight.

DISCLOSURE

The authors have nothing to disclose.

REFERENCES

1. Francis SA, Barnett N, Denham M. Switching of prescription drugs to over-the-counter status: is it a good thing for the elderly? Drugs Aging 2005;22(5): 361–70.

2. Administration USFaD. Drug applications for over-the-counter (OTC) drugs 2020. Available at: https://www.fda.gov/drugs/types-applications/drug-applications-over-counter-otc-drugs. Accessed 23 May, 2021.

3. OTC Use Statstics. Consumer healthcare products association 2021. Available at: https://chpa.org/about-consumer-healthcare/research-data/otc-use-statistics. Accessed 30 May, 2021.

4. Eng M. Potentially inappropriate OTC medications in older adults. US Pharmacist 2008;33(6):29–36.

5. American geriatrics society updated beers criteria for potentially inappropriate medication use in older adults. J Am Geriatr Soc 2012;60(4):616–31.

6. Sudano I, Flammer AJ, Roas S, et al. Nonsteroidal antiinflammatory drugs, acetaminophen, and hypertension. Curr Hypertens Rep 2012;14(4):304–9.

7. Griffin MR, Yared A, Ray WA. Nonsteroidal antiinflammatory drugs and acute renal failure in elderly persons. Am J Epidemiol 2000;151(5):488–96.

8. Beers MH. Explicit criteria for determining potentially inappropriate medication use by the elderly. An update. Arch Intern Med 1997;157(14):1531–6.

9. Fick DM, Cooper JW, Wade WE, et al. Updating the beers criteria for potentially inappropriate medication use in older adults: results of a US consensus panel of experts. Arch Intern Med 2003;163(22):2716–24.

10. O'Mahony D, O'Sullivan D, Byrne S, et al. STOPP/START criteria for potentially inappropriate prescribing in older people: version 2. Age Ageing 2015;44(2):213–8.

11. Weng MC, Tsai CF, Sheu KL, et al. The impact of number of drugs prescribed on the risk of potentially inappropriate medication among outpatient older adults with chronic diseases. QJM 2013;106(11):1009–15.

12. Qato DM, Wilder J, Schumm LP, et al. Changes in prescription and over-the-counter medication and dietary supplement use among older adults in the United States, 2005 vs 2011. JAMA Intern Med 2016;176(4):473–82.

13. Malec M, Shega JW. Pain management in the elderly. The Med Clin North America 2015;99(2):337–50.

14. Bear MD, Bartlett D, Evans P. Pharmacist counseling and the use of nonsteroidal anti-inflammatory drugs by older adults. Consult Pharm 2017;32(3):161–8.

15. Patel J, Ladani A, Sambamoorthi N, et al. A machine learning approach to identify predictors of potentially inappropriate non-steroidal anti-inflammatory drugs (NSAIDs) use in older adults with osteoarthritis. Int J Environ Res Public Health 2021;18(1):155.

16. Lind KE, Raban MZ, Georgiou A, et al. NSAID use among residents in 68 residential aged care facilities 2014 to 2017: an analysis of duration, concomitant medication use, and high-risk conditions. Pharmacoepidemiol Drug Saf 2019;28(11):1480–8.

17. Ford K, Whiting SJ. Vitamin and mineral supplement use by community-dwelling adults living in Canada and the United States: a scoping review. J Diet Suppl 2018;15(4):419–30.

18. Albert SM, Roth T, Toscani M, et al. Sleep health and appropriate use of OTC sleep aids in older adults-recommendations of a gerontological society of America workgroup. Gerontologist 2017;57(2):163–70.

19. Holden RJ, Srinivas P, Campbell NL, et al. Understanding older adults' medication decision making and behavior: a study on over-the-counter (OTC) anticholinergic medications. Res Social Adm Pharm 2019;15(1):53–60.

20. Kemper RF, Steiner V, Hicks B, et al. Anticholinergic medications: use among older adults with memory problems. J Gerontol Nurs 2007;33(1):21–9 [quiz 21–30].
21. Gross HJ, O'Neill G, Toscani M, et al. Sex differences in over-the-counter sleep aid use in older adults. Value Health 2015;18(3):A286–7.
22. Abraham O, Pu J, Schleiden LJ, et al. Factors contributing to poor satisfaction with sleep and healthcare seeking behavior in older adults. Sleep Health 2017;3(1):43–8.
23. Maust DT, Solway E, Clark SJ, et al. Prescription and nonprescription sleep product use among older adults in the United States. Am J Geriatr Psychiatry 2019;27(1):32–41.
24. American geriatrics society 2015 updated beers criteria for potentially inappropriate medication use in older adults. J Am Geriatr Soc 2015;63(11):2227–46.
25. Bharucha AE, Pemberton JH, Locke GR 3rd. American Gastroenterological Association technical review on constipation. Gastroenterology 2013;144(1): 218–38.
26. Gallegos-Orozco JF, Foxx-Orenstein AE, Sterler SM, et al. Chronic constipation in the elderly. Am J Gastroenterol 2012;107(1):18–25 [quiz 26].
27. Mugie SM, Benninga MA, Di Lorenzo C. Epidemiology of constipation in children and adults: a systematic review. Best Pract Res Clin Gastroenterol 2011; 25(1):3–18.
28. Bharucha AE, Zinsmeister AR, Locke GR, et al. Risk factors for fecal incontinence: a population-based study in women. Am J Gastroenterol 2006;101(6): 1305–12.
29. Bouras EP, Tangalos EG. Chronic constipation in the elderly. Gastroenterol Clin North Am 2009;38(3):463–80.
30. Werth BL, Christopher SA. Laxative use in the community: a literature review. J Clin Med 2021;10(1):143.
31. Goh LY, Vitry AI, Semple SJ, et al. Self-medication with over-the-counter drugs and complementary medications in South Australia's elderly population. BMC Complement Altern Med 2009;9:42.
32. Sheikh-Taha M, Dimassi H. Use of over the counter products in older cardiovascular patients admitted to a tertiary care center in USA. BMC Geriatr 2018; 18(1):301.
33. AlMutairi H, O'Dwyer M, Burke E, et al. Laxative use among older adults with intellectual disability: a cross-sectional observational study. Int J Clin Pharm 2020; 42(1):89–99.
34. Bailey RL, Gahche JJ, Miller PE, et al. Why US adults use dietary supplements. JAMA Intern Med 2013;173(5):355–61.
35. Gahche JJ, Bailey RL, Potischman N, et al. Dietary supplement use was very high among older adults in the United States in 2011-2014. J Nutr 2017; 147(10):1968–76.
36. Kurt M, Akdeniz M, Kavukcu E. Assessment of comorbidity and use of prescription and nonprescription drugs in patients above 65 Years attending family medicine outpatient clinics. Gerontol Geriatr Med 2019;5. 2333721419874274.
37. Eisenberg DM, Kessler RC, Foster C, et al. Unconventional medicine in the United States. Prevalence, costs, and patterns of use. N Engl J Med 1993; 328(4):246–52.
38. Eisenberg DM, Davis RB, Ettner SL, et al. Trends in alternative medicine use in the United States, 1990-1997: results of a follow-up national survey. JAMA 1998; 280(18):1569–75.

39. Zeilmann CA, Dole EJ, Skipper BJ, et al. Use of herbal medicine by elderly hispanic and non-hispanic white patients. Pharmacotherapy 2003;23(4):526–32.

40. González-Stuart A. Herbal product use by older adults. Maturitas 2011; 68(1):52–5.

41. Rashrash M, Schommer JC, Brown LM. Prevalence and predictors of herbal medicine use among adults in the United States. J Patient Exp 2017;4(3): 108–13.

42. Groden SR, Woodward AT, Chatters LM, et al. Use of complementary and alternative medicine among older adults: differences between baby boomers and pre-boomers. Am J Geriatr Psychiatry 2017;25(12):1393–401.

43. Dickinson A, MacKay D. Health habits and other characteristics of dietary supplement users: a review. Nutr J 2014;13:14.

44. Ylä-Rautio H, Siissalo S, Leikola S. Drug-related problems and pharmacy interventions in non-prescription medication, with a focus on high-risk over-the-counter medications. Int J Clin Pharm 2020;42(2):786–95.

45. Fielding S, Slovic P, Johnston M, et al. Public risk perception of non-prescription medicines and information disclosure during consultations: a suitable target for intervention? Int J Pharm Pract 2018;26(5):423–32.

46. Stone JA, Lester CA, Aboneh EA, et al. A preliminary examination of over-the-counter medication misuse rates in older adults. Res Social Adm Pharm 2017; 13(1):187–92.

47. Ramachandran A, Jaeschke H. Acetaminophen hepatotoxicity. Semin Liver Dis 2019;39(2):221–34.

48. Pharmacological management of persistent pain in older persons. J Am Geriatr Soc 2009;57(8):1331–46.

49. Schlondorff D. Renal complications of nonsteroidal anti-inflammatory drugs. Kidney Int 1993;44(3):643–53.

50. Harirforoosh S, Asghar W, Jamali F. Adverse effects of nonsteroidal antiinflammatory drugs: an update of gastrointestinal, cardiovascular and renal complications. J Pharm Pharm Sci 2013;16(5):821–47.

51. Wongrakpanich S, Wongrakpanich A, Melhado K, et al. A comprehensive review of non-steroidal anti-inflammatory drug use in the elderly. Aging Dis 2018;9(1): 143–50.

52. Cheng Y, Austin SC, Rocca B, et al. Role of prostacyclin in the cardiovascular response to thromboxane A2. Science 2002;296(5567):539–41.

53. Mallet L, Kuyumjian J. Indomethacin-induced behavioral changes in an elderly patient with dementia. Ann Pharmacother 1998;32(2):201–3.

54. Ochs KL, Zell-Kanter M, Mycyk MB. Hot, blind, and mad: avoidable geriatric anticholinergic delirium. Am J Emerg Med 2012;30(3):514, e511–3.

55. Ford AC, Moayyedi P, Lacy BE, et al. American College of Gastroenterology monograph on the management of irritable bowel syndrome and chronic idiopathic constipation. Am J Gastroenterol 2014;109(Suppl 1):S2–26 [quiz S27].

56. Brandt LJ, Prather CM, Quigley EM, et al. Systematic review on the management of chronic constipation in North America. Am J Gastroenterol 2005; 100(Suppl 1):S5–21.

57. Ford AC, Suares NC. Effect of laxatives and pharmacological therapies in chronic idiopathic constipation: systematic review and meta-analysis. Gut 2011;60(2):209–18.

58. Kamel NS, Gammack JK. Insomnia in the elderly: cause, approach, and treatment. Am J Med 2006;119(6):463–9.

59. Hutchison LC, O'Brien CE. Changes in pharmacokinetics and pharmacody-namics in the elderly patient. J Pharm Pract 2007;20(1):4–12.
60. Woodward M. Hypnosedatives in the elderly. CNS Drugs 1999;11(4):263–79.
61. Ishitsuka Y, Kondo Y, Kadowaki D. Toxicological property of acetaminophen: the dark side of a safe antipyretic/analgesic drug? Biol Pharm Bull 2020;43(2): 195–206.
62. Sekhar RV, Patel SG, Guthikonda AP, et al. Deficient synthesis of glutathione un-derlies oxidative stress in aging and can be corrected by dietary cysteine and glycine supplementation. Am J Clin Nutr 2011;94(3):847–53.
63. Suh JH, Wang H, Liu RM, et al. (R)-alpha-lipoic acid reverses the age-related loss in GSH redox status in post-mitotic tissues: evidence for increased cysteine requirement for GSH synthesis. Arch Biochem Biophys 2004;423(1):126–35.
64. Ali A, Arif AW, Bhan C, et al. Managing chronic pain in the elderly: an overview of the recent therapeutic advancements. Cureus 2018;10(9):e3293.
65. Cryer B, Feldman M. Cyclooxygenase-1 and cyclooxygenase-2 selectivity of widely used nonsteroidal anti-inflammatory drugs. Am J Med 1998;104(5): 413–21.
66. Laine L, Curtis SP, Cryer B, et al. Risk factors for NSAID-associated upper GI clinical events in a long-term prospective study of 34 701 arthritis patients. Aliment Pharmacol Ther 2010;32(10):1240–8.
67. Carro A, Kaski JC. Myocardial infarction in the elderly. Aging Dis 2011;2(2): 116–37.
68. Gooch K, Culleton BF, Manns BJ, et al. NSAID use and progression of chronic kidney disease. Am J Med 2007;120(3):280, e281–7.
69. Rickels K, Morris RJ, Newman H, et al. Diphenhydramine in insomniac family practice patients: a double-blind study. J Clin Pharmacol 1983;23(5–6):234–42.
70. Glass JR, Sproule BA, Herrmann N, et al. Effects of 2-week treatment with tema-zepam and diphenhydramine in elderly insomniacs: a randomized, placebo-controlled trial. J Clin Psychopharmacol 2008;28(2):182–8.
71. McEvoy LK, Smith ME, Fordyce M, et al. Characterizing impaired functional alertness from diphenhydramine in the elderly with performance and neuro-physiologic measures. Sleep 2006;29(7):957–66.
72. Morin CM, Koetter U, Bastien C, et al. Valerian-hops combination and diphenhy-dramine for treating insomnia: a randomized placebo-controlled clinical trial. Sleep 2005;28(11):1465–71.
73. Agostini JV, Leo-Summers LS, Inouye SK. Cognitive and other adverse effects of diphenhydramine use in hospitalized older patients. Arch Intern Med 2001; 161(17):2091–7.
74. Vazquez Roque M, Bouras EP. Epidemiology and management of chronic con-stipation in elderly patients. Clin interventions Aging 2015;10:919–30.
75. Suares NC, Ford AC. Systematic review: the effects of fibre in the management of chronic idiopathic constipation. Aliment Pharmacol Ther 2011;33(8):895–901.
76. Mounsey A, Raleigh M, Wilson A. Management of constipation in older adults. Am Fam Physician 2015;92(6):500–4.
77. Ramkumar D, Rao SS. Efficacy and safety of traditional medical therapies for chronic constipation: systematic review. Am J Gastroenterol 2005;100(4): 936–71.
78. Harris LA, Horn J, Kissous-Hunt M, et al. The better understanding and recog-nition of the disconnects, experiences, and needs of patients with chronic idio-pathic constipation (BURDEN-CIC) study: results of an online questionnaire. Adv Ther 2017;34(12):2661–73.

79. Nyberg C, Hendel J, Nielsen OH. The safety of osmotically acting cathartics in colonic cleansing. Nat Rev Gastroenterol Hepatol 2010;7(10):557–64.

80. Antolin-Amerigo D, Sánchez-González MJ, Barbarroja-Escudero J, et al. Allergic reaction to polyethylene glycol in a painter. Occup Med 2015;65(6): 502–4.

81. Hurst FP, Bohen EM, Osgard EM, et al. Association of oral sodium phosphate purgative use with acute kidney injury. J Am Soc Nephrol 2007;18(12):3192–8.

82. Curhan GC, Willett WC, Speizer FE, et al. Comparison of dietary calcium with supplemental calcium and other nutrients as factors affecting the risk for kidney stones in women. Ann Intern Med 1997;126(7):497–504.

83. Marriott BM. Vitamin D supplementation: a word of caution. Ann Intern Med 1997;127(3):231–3.

84. Molinari M, Watt KD, Kruszyna T, et al. Acute liver failure induced by green tea extracts: case report and review of the literature. Liver Transpl 2006;12(12): 1892–5.

85. Bent S, Goldberg H, Padula A, et al. Spontaneous bleeding associated with ginkgo biloba: a case report and systematic review of the literature: a case report and systematic review of the literature. J Gen Intern Med 2005;20(7): 657–61.

86. Matthews MK Jr. Association of Ginkgo biloba with intracerebral hemorrhage. Neurology 1998;50(6):1933–4.

87. Stoddard GJ, Archer M, Shane-McWhorter L, et al. Ginkgo and warfarin interaction in a large veterans administration population. AMIA Annu Symp Proc 2015; 2015:1174–83.

88. Engelsen J, Nielsen JD, Winther K. Effect of coenzyme Q10 and Ginkgo biloba on warfarin dosage in stable, long-term warfarin treated outpatients. A randomised, double blind, placebo-crossover trial. Thromb Haemost 2002;87(6): 1075–6.

89. Köhler S, Funk P, Kieser M. Influence of a 7-day treatment with Ginkgo biloba special extract EGb 761 on bleeding time and coagulation: a randomized, placebo-controlled, double-blind study in healthy volunteers. Blood Coagul Fibrinolysis 2004;15(4):303–9.

90. Jiang X, Williams KM, Liauw WS, et al. Effect of ginkgo and ginger on the pharmacokinetics and pharmacodynamics of warfarin in healthy subjects. Br J Clin Pharmacol 2005;59(4):425–32.

91. Izzo AA, Hoon-Kim S, Radhakrishnan R, et al. A critical approach to evaluating clinical efficacy, adverse events and drug interactions of herbal remedies. Phytother Res 2016;30(5):691–700.

92. Malati CY, Robertson SM, Hunt JD, et al. Influence of Panax ginseng on cytochrome P450 (CYP)3A and P-glycoprotein (P-gp) activity in healthy participants. J Clin Pharmacol 2012;52(6):932–9.

93. Jiang X, Williams KM, Liauw WS, et al. Effect of St John's wort and ginseng on the pharmacokinetics and pharmacodynamics of warfarin in healthy subjects. Br J Clin Pharmacol 2004;57(5):592–9.

94. Mueller SC, Uehleke B, Woehling H, et al. Effect of St John's wort dose and preparations on the pharmacokinetics of digoxin. Clin Pharmacol Ther 2004;75(6): 546–57.

95. Lantz MS, Buchalter E, Giambanco V. St. John's wort and antidepressant drug interactions in the elderly. J Geriatr Psychiatry Neurol 1999;12(1):7–10.

96. Pastori D, Carnevale R, Cangemi R, et al. Vitamin E serum levels and bleeding risk in patients receiving oral anticoagulant therapy: a retrospective cohort study. J Am Heart Assoc 2013;2(6):e000364.

97. Williams CT. Herbal supplements: precautions and safe use. Nurs Clin North Am 2021;56(1):1–21.

98. Kellermann AJ, Kloft C. Is there a risk of bleeding associated with standardized Ginkgo biloba extract therapy? A systematic review and meta-analysis. Pharmacotherapy 2011;31(5):490–502.

99. Moore N, Pollack C, Butkerait P. Adverse drug reactions and drug-drug interactions with over-the-counter NSAIDs. Ther Clin Risk Manag 2015;11:1061–75.

100. Kim J, Parish AL. Polypharmacy and medication management in older adults. Nurs Clin North Am 2017;52(3):457–68.

101. Jokanovic N, Tan EC, Dooley MJ, et al. Prevalence and factors associated with polypharmacy in long-term care facilities: a systematic review. J Am Med Dir Assoc 2015;16(6):535, e531–512.

102. Morin L, Vetrano DL, Rizzuto D, et al. Choosing wisely? Measuring the burden of medications in older adults near the end of life: nationwide, longitudinal cohort study. Am J Med 2017;130(8):927–36.e9.

103. Farrell DKB. Polypharmacy: optimizing medication use in elderly patients. Pharm Pract 2014;20–5.

104. Liu Y, Ramírez J, Ratain MJ. Inhibition of paracetamol glucuronidation by tyrosine kinase inhibitors. Br J Clin Pharmacol 2011;71(6):917–20.

105. Savina PM, Brouwer KL. Probenecid-impaired biliary excretion of acetaminophen glucuronide and sulfate in the rat. Drug Metab Dispos 1992;20(4):496–501.

106. Kostrubsky SE, Sinclair JF, Strom SC, et al. Phenobarbital and phenytoin increased acetaminophen hepatotoxicity due to inhibition of UDP-glucuronosyltransferases in cultured human hepatocytes. Toxicol Sci 2005;87(1):146–55.

107. Jickling G, Heino A, Ahmed SN. Acetaminophen toxicity with concomitant use of carbamazepine. Epileptic Disord 2009;11(4):329–32.

108. Nassar I, Pasupati T, Judson JP, et al. Reduced exposure of imatinib after coadministration with acetaminophen in mice. Indian J Pharmacol 2009;41(4):167–72.

109. Gastrup S, Stage TB, Fruekilde PB, et al. Paracetamol decreases steady-state exposure to lamotrigine by induction of glucuronidation in healthy subjects. Br J Clin Pharmacol 2016;81(4):735–41.

110. Galinsky RE, Nelson EB, Rollins DE. Pharmacokinetic consequences and toxicologic implications of metyrapone-induced alterations of acetaminophen elimination in man. Eur J Clin Pharmacol 1987;33(4):391–6.

111. Atkinson HC, Stanescu I, Salem I, et al. Increased bioavailability of phenylephrine by co-administration of acetaminophen: results of four open-label, crossover pharmacokinetic trials in healthy volunteers. Eur J Clin Pharmacol 2015;71(2):151–8.

112. Dimova S, Stoytchev T. Influence of rifampicin on the toxicity and the analgesic effect of acetaminophen. Eur J Drug Metab Pharmacokinet 1994;19(4):311–7.

113. Gebauer MG, Nyfort-Hansen K, Henschke PJ, et al. Warfarin and acetaminophen interaction. Pharmacotherapy 2003;23(1):109–12.

114. Abdulla A, Adams N, Bone M, et al. Guidance on the management of pain in older people. Age Ageing 2013;42(Suppl 1):i1–57.

115. Huynh DA, Abbas M, Dabaja A. Diphenhydramine toxicity. In: StatPearls. Treasure Island (FL): StatPearls Publishing Copyright © 2021, StatPearls Publishing LLC; 2021.

116. Markowitz JS, Donovan JL, DeVane CL, et al. Effect of St John's wort on drug metabolism by induction of cytochrome P450 3A4 enzyme. JAMA 2003; 290(11):1500–4.

117. Uesawa Y, Takeuchi T, Mohri K. Integrated analysis on the physicochemical properties of dihydropyridine calcium channel blockers in grapefruit juice interactions. Curr Pharm Biotechnol 2012;13(9):1705–17.

118. Mouly S, Lloret-Linares C, Sellier PO, et al. Is the clinical relevance of drug-food and drug-herb interactions limited to grapefruit juice and Saint-John's Wort? Pharmacol Res 2017;118:82–92.

119. Radandt JM, Marchbanks CR, Dudley MN. Interactions of fluoroquinolones with other drugs: mechanisms, variability, clinical significance, and management. Clin Infect Dis 1992;14(1):272–84.

120. Wimbiscus M, Kostenko O, Malone D. MAO inhibitors: risks, benefits, and lore. Cleve Clin J Med 2010;77(12):859–82.

121. Public Law No: 116-136 (03/27/2020), Available at: https://www.congress.gov/bill/116th-congress/house-bill/748. Accessed August 27, 2021.

122. Register USGOotF. Title 21, chapter 1, subchapter D: drugs for human use. Office of the federal register. Code of federal regulations; 2021. Available at: https://www.ecfr.gov/cgi-bin/text-idx?SID=004162a80667cb41246e45477e4a 16ad&mc=true&tpl=/ecfrbrowse/Title21/21cfrv5_02.tpl#0. Accessed 22 May, 2021.

123. Administration USFaD. Over-the-Counter OTC nonprescription drugs. United States Government; 2020. Available at: https://www.fda.gov/drugs/how-drugs-are-developed-and-approved/over-counter-otc-nonprescription-drugs. Accessed 22 May, 2021.

124. Congress U. S.784 - dietary supplement health and education act of 1994. Available at: https://www.congress.gov/bill/103rd-congress/senate-bill/784. Accessed 5 May, 2021.

125. Hamburg MA, Letter from commissioner of food and drugs to manufacturers of dietary supplements. Available at: http://www.fda.gov/downloads/Drugs/Resources ForYou/Consumers/BuyingUsingMedicineSafely/MedicationHealthFraud/UCM236 985.pdf. Accessed August 27, 2021.

126. Sarma N, Giancaspro G, Venema J. Dietary supplements quality analysis tools from the United States Pharmacopeia. Drug Test Anal 2016;8(3–4):418–23.

127. Administration FaD. MedWatch online voluntary reporting form. U. S. Food & Drug Administration; 2021. Available at: https://www.accessdata.fda.gov/scripts/medwatch/. Accessed 15 May, 2021.

128. Holmes JL, Biella A, Morck T, et al. Medical foods: science, regulation, and practical aspects. Summary of a workshop. Curr Dev Nutr 2021;5(Suppl 1):nzaa172.

129. Is it really FDA approved? Food and drug administration; 2017. Available at: https://www.fda.gov/consumers/consumer-updates/it-really-fda-approved. Accessed 15 May, 2021.

130. Agarwal E, Marshall S, Miller M, et al. Optimising nutrition in residential aged care: a narrative review. Maturitas 2016;92:70–8.

131. Bruins MJ, Van Dael P, Eggersdorfer M. The role of nutrients in reducing the risk for noncommunicable diseases during aging. Nutrients 2019;11(1):85.

132. Commission FT. Dietary supplements: an advertising guide for industry. Federal Trade Commission; 2001. Available at: https://www.ftc.gov/tips-advice/business-center/guidance/dietary-supplements-advertising-guide-industry. Accessed August 27, 2021.

133. Commission FT. Enforcement policy statement on food advertising. In: Commission FT, ed 1994. Available at: https://www.ftc.gov/public-statements/1994/05/enforcement-policy-statement-food-advertising. Accessed August 27, 2021.

134. Heyman ML, Williams RL. Ensuring global access to quality medicines: role of the US Pharmacopeia. J Pharm Sci 2011;100(4):1280–7.

135. Straub DA. Calcium supplementation in clinical practice: a review of forms, doses, and indications. Nutr Clin Pract 2007;22(3):286–96.

136. Convention TUSP. Verification services. 2021. Available at: https://www.usp.org/services/verification-services. Accessed 15 May, 2021.

137. Convention TUSP. USP verified dietary supplements 2021. Available at: https://www.quality-supplements.org/verified-products. Accessed 15 May, 2021.

138. Australian regulatory guidelines for listed medicines and registered complementary medicines. Therapeutic Goods Administration; 2020. Available at: https://www.tga.gov.au/publication/australian-regulatory-guidelines-listed-medicines-and-registered-complementary-medicines. Accessed 15 May, 2021.

139. Thakkar S, Anklam E, Xu A, et al. Regulatory landscape of dietary supplements and herbal medicines from a global perspective. Regul Toxicol Pharmacol 2020;114:104647.

140. Dwyer JT, Coates PM, Smith MJ. Dietary supplements: regulatory challenges and research resources. Nutrients 2018;10(1):41.

141. Albert SM, Bix L, Bridgeman MM, et al. Promoting safe and effective use of OTC medications: CHPA-GSA National Summit. Gerontologist 2014;54(6):909–18.

142. Klein-Schwartz W, Oderda GM. Poisoning in the elderly. Epidemiological, clinical and management considerations. Drugs Aging 1991;1(1):67–89.

143. Administration USFaD. Tips for older dietary supplement users. U.S. Food and Drug Administration; 2017. Available at: https://www.fda.gov/food/information-consumers-using-dietary-supplements/tips-older-dietary-supplement-users. Accessed 23 May, 2021.

144. Berkman ND, Sheridan SL, Donahue KE, et al. Health literacy interventions and outcomes: an updated systematic review. Evid Rep Technol Assess 2011;199:1–941.

145. Administration USFaD. The over-the-counter medication label: take a look. U.S. Food and Drug Administration; 2017. Available at: https://www.fda.gov/drugs/resources-you-drugs/over-counter-medicine-label-take-look. Accessed 23 May, 2021.

146. Roumie CL, Griffin MR. Over-the-counter analgesics in older adults: a call for improved labelling and consumer education. Drugs Aging 2004;21(8):485–98.

147. Raghavan A, Paliwal Y, Slattum PW. Gaps in OTC labeling: potentially inappropriate medications for older adults. Consult Pharm 2018;33(3):159–62.

148. Mrvos R, Dean BS, Krenzelok EP. Illiteracy: a contributing factor to poisoning. Vet Hum Toxicol 1993;35(5):466–8.

149. Mansoor LE, Dowse R. Effect of pictograms on readability of patient information materials. Ann Pharmacother 2003;37(7–8):1003–9.

150. Jariangprasert CS, El-Ibiary SY, Tsourounis C, et al. What women want to know: an assessment of online questions asked by women using an ask-the-pharmacist service. J Pharm Technol 2007;23(4):214–20.

151. Health Communication and Health Information Technology. Office of disease prevention and health promotion 2021. Available at: http://www.healthypeople.gov/2020/topicsobjectives2020/overview.aspx?topicid=18. Accessed 24 May, 2021.

152. Martin-Hammond AM, Abegaz T, Gilbert JE. Designing an over-the-counter consumer decision-making tool for older adults. J Biomed Inform 2015;57:113–23.

153. Holden MD. Over-the-counter medications. Do you know what your patients are taking? Postgrad Med 1992;91(8):191–4, 199–200.

154. Honig PK, Gillespie BK. Drug interactions between prescribed and over-the-counter medication. Drug Saf 1995;13(5):296–303.

155. Honig PK, Gillespie BK. Clinical significance of pharmacokinetic drug interactions with over-the-counter (OTC) drugs. Clin Pharmacokinet 1998;35(3):167–71.

156. Sleath B, Rubin RH, Campbell W, et al. Physician-patient communication about over-the-counter medications. Soc Sci Med 2001;53(3):357–69.

157. Phillips LA, Leventhal H, Leventhal EA. Physicians' communication of the common-sense self-regulation model results in greater reported adherence than physicians' use of interpersonal skills. Br J Health Psychol 2012;17(2):244–57.

158. Resources for health care providers. NIH national center for complementary and Integrative health. Available at: https://www.fda.gov/food/information-consumers-using-dietary-supplements/tips-older-dietary-supplement-users. Accessed 23 May, 2021.

159. How safe is this product or practice? NIH national center for complementary and Integrative health. Available at: https://www.nccih.nih.gov/health/how-safe-is-this-product-or-practice. Accessed 23 May, 2021.

160. Singh M, Short D, Manzie J, et al. Impact of medical education program on HCPs and patient understanding of COPD (joint working with GSK). Eur Respir J 2014;44(Suppl 58):P2802.

161. Henley E, Wenzel-Wamhoff J. Teaching medical students about over-the-counter medications. Med Educ 2000;34(7):580–2.

162. Cohen PA. The FDA and adulterated supplements—dereliction of duty. JAMA Netw Open 2018;1(6):e183329.

163. Supplements NIoHOoD. Dietary supplement label database. National Institutes of Health Office of Dietary Supplements; 2013. Available at: https://ods.od.nih.gov/Research/Dietary_Supplement_Label_Database.aspx. Accessed 20 May, 2021.

164. Supplements NIfHOoD. Dietary supplement ingredient database 2017. Available at: https://dsid.od.nih.gov/. Accessed 20 May, 2021.

165. Abernethy D, Sheehan C, Griffiths J, et al. Adulteration of drugs and foods: compendial approaches to lowering risk. Clin Pharmacol Ther 2009;85(4):444–7.

Nicotine Use Disorder in Older Adults

Nazem K. Bassil, MD[a],*, Marie Lena K. Ohanian, MD[b], Theodora G. Bou Saba, MD[b]

KEYWORDS

- Nicotine abuse • Elderly • Smoking cessation

KEY POINTS

- Nicotine use disorder is a common problem in the elderly.
- The older adult should fulfill at least 2 out the 11 criteria in the *Diagnostic and Statistical Manual of Mental Disorders* (Fifth Edition) to be considered a nicotine misuser.
- Smoking in the elderly is associated with anxiety, depression, and low socioeconomic status.
- It is mostly a habit, and some find pleasure in smoking; thus, cessation in the elderly is a difficult task.
- Smoking has a detrimental effect on several organ systems; many problems manifest in the older age group.

INTRODUCTION

"I've been enjoying cigarettes for many decades, and the damage has already been done."[1] This is one common statement made by older adults when asked about their intention to stop smoking.

Tobacco use is a worldwide problem affecting all age groups, and one of the leading causes of morbidity and mortality. Nicotine is among the most psychoactive drug used. Usually, people try it for the first time in the form of cigarettes, hubble-bubbles, e-cigarettes, pipe, or similar at a younger age; therefore, many doctors and scientists think that nicotine use disorder is a younger-generation issue.

Many older adults try to quit; some succeed, and others do not.[2] One of the main reasons for smoking cessation is that older adults are more prone to develop health problems related to the cumulative effect of smoking. Stopping smoking at any age can promote longevity and improve the quality of life.[2] However, giving up smoking is a difficult task in the older population because of several factors. First, tobacco

[a] Geriatric Medicine, Palliative Care, Balamand University, Saint George Hospital University Medical Center, Beirut, Lebanon; [b] Family Medicine, Balamand University, Saint George Hospital University Medical Center, Beirut, Lebanon
* Corresponding author.
E-mail address: bassilnazem@gmail.com

Clin Geriatr Med 38 (2022) 119–131
https://doi.org/10.1016/j.cger.2021.07.008
0749-0690/22/© 2021 Elsevier Inc. All rights reserved.

use disorder is acquired since adolescence/younger adulthood; hence, it is difficult for them to quit smoking. Furthermore, some older people have poor insight about the harm of tobacco consumption. Thus, enters the role of physicians in counseling and assisting smokers in quitting by offering nicotine replacement therapy or other modalities.[2]

DEFINITION OF NICOTINE USE DISORDER

Nicotine use disorder, also known as tobacco use disorder, is defined as the problematic use of tobacco leading to a significant impairment and distress in a person's everyday life. The patient should at least fulfill 2 out of the 11 criteria defined by the *Diagnostic and Statistical Manual of Mental Disorders* (Fifth Edition) that should be occurring within a 12-month period to be considered a tobacco misuser. These criteria mainly involve the amount and time spent on smoking, the constant desire for smoking, the inability to stop, and the interference of smoking with daily life activities on the social and occupational levels[3] (**Box 1**).

In contrast to the adult population, certain considerations should be accounted for in older adults. For instance, cognitive impairment can prevent adequate self-monitoring. In addition, symptoms of nicotine use disorder can occur with a smaller amount of nicotine consumed. Also, role obligations may be reduced in older adults. Certain seniors may not be aware of the problems that they experience from tobacco use.

Older adults may experience more severe symptoms from nicotine withdrawal, such as anxiety, restlessness, poor concentration, increased appetite, and insomnia. Older adults are at higher risk of adverse functional and cognitive complications associated with smoking cessation compared with the middle-aged population. Finally, nicotine withdrawal, especially if acute, is associated with a higher risk of hyperactive delirium in patients with an underlying cognitive impairment.[3]

Prevalence

According to the 2019 Centers for Disease Control and Prevention (CDC) data, smoking is more common among young people (17%) compared with only 8.2% in the

---

Box 1
Diagnostic and Statistical Manual of Mental Disorders **(Fifth Edition) criteria for tobacco use disorder**

1. Smoking in higher amounts or over a longer period of time than intended.
2. Persistent need for smoking or inability to cut down tobacco use.
3. Large amount of time spent on activities to obtain tobacco.
4. Cravings.
5. Tobacco use interfering with the ability to fulfill major obligations.
6. Continued tobacco use despite social and interpersonal problems caused by smoking.
7. Reduced social and occupational activities because of smoking.
8. Tobacco use in situations that put the person at risk.
9. Tobacco use despite having physical and psychological problems caused by smoking.
10. Tolerance defined as the need to increase the amount to obtain the same effect.
11. Withdrawal defined by withdrawal symptoms (headaches, difficulty concentrating, nervousness, insomnia) and the need to use similar products.

elderly.[4] Nonetheless, contradictory data show that older people are less likely to quit smoking than their younger counterparts. Furthermore, between 1965 and 1994, smoking rates dropped less in patients aged more than 65 years (5.9% reduction) than in younger adults (18.4% reduction).[4] Also, the absolute number of older smokers is anticipated to double in 2050,[4] with the aging of baby boomers.[5] In Europe, the prevalence of smoking is high (21.9%), mainly in the age group between 25 and 54 years (83% of the smoking population). In the older age groups, the prevalence is 12.2% in men between the age of 65 and 74 years and 8.4% among women of the same age group.[6]

Risk Factors

Concerning the risk factors for smoking (**Box 2**), it was found that nicotine use disorder was more prevalent in the elderly with low socioeconomic status, alcohol use disorder, anxiety, and depression. Moreover, stress was associated with substance abuse in the elderly. In fact, at the end of life, many stressors can be found that can incite the aging patient to adhere to old habits that make them comfortable, such as smoking (**Box 3**).[7,8]

A study done in Australia in 1999 by Degenhardt and colleagues[9] showed that alcohol, cannabis, and other drug use disorders were significantly more common among current smokers, supporting the findings of previous studies. Furthermore, a study done in hospitalized patients with chronic obstructive pulmonary disease (COPD) showed that 45% of the smokers still smoked and did not understand or accept the dangerous effects of tobacco as a reason they refused to quit smoking.[10]

Pleasure and Social Interactions

Many older adults report that they started smoking in their youth, because of peer pressure and the need to be accepted socially by their friends who smoked and be part of a group, not because of pleasure in smoking. Because of the increased nicotinic receptors in the brain and the increased secretion of endorphins, the older adult will find pleasure in smoking, and reduction of anxiety and stress. However, many of long-time older smokers will state that little pleasure results from smoking compared with when they were younger.[2] For many, it has been a part of their social life, and this is observed well with the hubble-bubble, where some gather to smoke.

Habit of Smoking

Many older adults integrated smoking in their daily life routine. They smoke before going to the bathroom, after meals, with coffee, with alcohol, with stress, and with happiness.[2]

Box 2
Risk factors for smoking in the elderly
Low socioeconomic status
Alcohol use disorder
Psychiatric comorbidities (anxiety, depression, and so forth)
Life stressors

Box 3
Life stressors contributing to tobacco use in the elderly

Personal illness: 18%

Decline in the 5 senses (and decline of physical reserve)

Illness at home: 23%

Nonmedical event: 17% (familial conflicts)

Family changes

Retirement

Change in income

Communication problems

EFFECTS OF SMOKING ON HEALTH

Smoking is established as being the most preventable cause of mortality. It is considered one of the major risk factors for the development of chronic diseases, including cardiovascular, respiratory system, eyes, gums, and bones, that can have debilitating consequences on the elderly. It is also associated with increased risk of cancer. Because of the additive effect of nicotine and harmful substances found in cigarettes, deleterious health effects are more commonly seen in the elderly than in the younger population[11] (**Box 4**).

Smoking remains a strong risk factor for premature mortality in older age groups.[12]

Smoking and Cardiovascular Diseases

Cardiovascular diseases (CVD) are the leading cause of death in both men and women, especially in the elderly population. Tobacco smoking is a major preventable risk factor for CVD, mainly coronary artery diseases (CAD).

Mortality from coronary heart disease is doubled in smokers compared with non-smokers.[9] Also, older smokers are at a higher risk of developing heart failure and its decompensation.

A study performed by Nadruz and colleagues[13] entitled, "Smoking and cardiac structure and function in the elderly," showed that smokers have a higher left ventricular mass, higher prevalence of left ventricular hypertrophy, a major risk factor for heart failure, and worse diastolic function compared with nonsmokers or former smokers. Left ventricular hypertrophy is a major risk factor for heart failure.

In addition, smoking increases baseline blood pressure and heart rate and reduces blood flow to the heart and oxygen delivery to the vital organs. It damages blood vessels, increases the risk of thrombosis, and doubles the risk of stroke.[14]

Furthermore, older smokers are at higher risk of developing arrhythmias, including atrial fibrillation. Smoking is also a major cause for the development of abdominal aortic aneurysms; according to the CDC, almost all deaths from abdominal aortic aneurysms are caused by smoking.[15]

Smoking is a known risk factor for strokes, both ischemic and hemorrhagic. Several studies showed that smokers have two- to fourfold increased risk of stroke compared with nonsmokers and former smokers. Stroke has a dose-dependent relationship with smoking.[11]

Box 4
Effects of smoking on health[2]

Cardiovascular diseases

Stroke

Coronary artery disease and congestive heart failure

Peripheral artery disease

Arrhythmias

Aortic aneurysms and dissection

Pulmonary and respiratory diseases

Chronic obstructive lung disease

Uncontrolled asthma

Lung fibrosis

Postoperative lung problems

Pulmonary hypertension

Pulmonary embolisms and deep vein thrombosis

Sinusitis

Cancer

Lung

Gastric

Head and neck

Bladder and kidney

Gastrointestinal

Peptic ulcer disease and gastroesophageal reflux

Bone: Osteoporosis

Skin

Poor wound healing

Skin aging and wrinkles

THE PATHOPHYSIOLOGY OF CIGARETTE SMOKING AND CARDIOVASCULAR DISEASE

Smoking affects all phases of atherosclerosis by increasing inflammation and decreasing nitric oxide and the low-density lipoproteins (LDL) oxidation. In fact, cigarette smoking decreases the vasodilation ability of the vessels by lowering the amount of nitric oxide, which is one of the early manifestations of atherosclerotic changes. In addition, smoking increases the peripheral blood leukocytes count and other inflammatory markers that deposit on the surface of endothelial cells and promotes atherosclerosis. Likewise, cigarette smoking increases serum lipid profile, mainly LDL, and leads to its oxidation, which promotes atherosclerosis and therefore increases the risk of CAD.[16] To note, smoking has a prothrombotic effect: it alters platelet functions and thrombotic and fibrinolytic factors. The atherosclerotic and prothrombotic effects of smoking increase the risk of acute cardiovascular events.[17]

Smoking and Respiratory Diseases

Smoking is responsible for 90% of cases of COPD and lung cancer deaths.[18]

In fact, it leads to the activation of epithelial cells, macrophages, and lymphocytes and to the loss of fibroblasts, which promotes the release of cytokines, growth factors, and matrix metalloproteinases, leading to lung remodeling.[13]

Also, smokers have a higher prevalence of COPD and a higher mortality. Besides knowing that aging is a risk factor for COPD, as lung capacity and function start to decline naturally within the fourth decade of life, smoking accelerates their destruction and predisposes them to more severe consequences.[13]

Tobacco is also an important risk factor for community-acquired pneumonia; it interferes with the ability of the respiratory system to clear bacteria by damaging the mucociliary clearance mechanism and modifying the buccal epithelial surfaces, making them at a higher risk for pneumococcal diseases. Smoking also increases the incidence, duration, and severity of respiratory infections caused by bacteria and viruses.[13]

Smoking is a major risk factor for postoperative pulmonary complications. A patient more than 60 years of age is already at risk for complications; smoking increases their risk for atelectasis and pneumonia.[13]

Smoking and Sinusitis

Sinusitis is one of the most prevalent health conditions worldwide, and a common complaint in the primary care clinics. The incidence of sinusitis increases in a dose-dependent manner with smoking. Sinonasal epithelial cells depend on the mucociliary clearance mechanism to clear potentially toxic substances, and that is inhibited by chemicals emitted from smoking, leading to stasis of these materials, increasing the risk of bacterial infections and subsequently sinusitis.[19]

Smoking and Cancer

According to the American Cancer Society,[20] smoking is responsible for about 20% of all cancers and 30% of all cancer deaths in the United States. It increases the risk mainly of mouth, larynx, pharynx, lungs, esophagus, kidney, cervix, liver, bladder, pancreas, stomach, and colon cancers. Lung cancer is among the most common cancers worldwide and the major cause of cancer deaths in developed countries. According to the CDC,[21] patients who smoke are 15 to 30 times more likely to have or to die from lung cancer than the nonsmoker. In fact, 80% of lung cancer cases are due to smoking. Oral cavity and oropharyngeal cancers are more common in smokers. The amount and the duration of smoking determine the risk of the development of such types of cancers.

Smoking and Osteoporosis

Smoking is a known risk factor for the development of osteoporosis, and several studies showed a direct association between smoking and low bone density. The National Institute of Osteoporosis reports that smoking increases the risk of fractures and has a bad impact on bone healing after fracture. Smoking also induces a faster menopause, which in turn may lead to a higher risk of osteoporosis.[22]

Smoking and Ophthalmic Diseases

With the aging population, the incidence of cataracts is increasing. Smoking is one of the risk factors that augments cataract development by threefold compared with nonsmokers.[23]

Furthermore, age-related macular degeneration, a major cause of blindness in developed countries in the elderly, is also affected by smoking.[24]

Smoking and Dermatologic Diseases

Several studies have showed the relationship between smoking and facial wrinkles, which are signs of aging. For instance, a study conducted by Leung and colleagues[25] showed that the skin's age is proportional to the time and duration of smoking. In older age, smoking a pack of cigarettes per day is the equivalent of several years of skin aging.

Smoking and Neuropsychiatric Disorders

Nicotine receptors in the brain

Nicotine binds mainly to nicotinic cholinergic receptors in the brain. This process leads to an increase in the activity of several brain regions, including the prefrontal cortex and the thalamus, and secretion of several neurotransmitters, including dopamine. This release is responsible for the pleasurable experience of cigarette smoking. With the continuous use of nicotine, an increased amount of nicotine is needed to exert the same effect. This is mainly explained by the process of tolerance caused by the desensitization of the receptors and the increase in the number of nicotine receptors in the brain. Smokers have a larger number of nicotine receptors in their brain than nonsmokers. Certain studies showed that smokers with a higher amount of nicotine receptors in their brain face more difficulty quitting because of cravings and more severe withdrawal symptoms.[26]

Effect on cognition

Smoking increases the risk of dementia, especially Alzheimer disease and vascular dementia, mainly because of vascular events, such as silent strokes, oxidative stress atherosclerosis, and inflammation.[27] The association with cognitive impairment might be due to the link between smoking and cardiovascular pathologic condition, but cigarette smoke also contains neurotoxins, which heighten the risk.[28] In fact, a study has shown that smoking is associated with decreased gray matter in regions associated with Alzheimer disease (medial temporal lobe structures, posterior cingulum, and precuneus).[29] Smoking is a modifiable risk factor for Alzheimer disease[30]; thus, smoking cessation might delay the development of Alzheimer disease.[31] Smoking in later life is also associated with 1.6 relative risk for dementia, with a weighed population attributable fraction risk of 5.5%.[32]

The British National Birth Cohort Study found that smokers had a greater decline in global memory, whereas their visual memory was preserved. The Doetinchem Study added that smokers have decreased cognitive flexibility, speed, and function. This study shows that the decline among smokers was 1.9 times higher in the memory function, 2.4 times higher in cognitive flexibility, and 1.7 times greater for global cognitive function compared with nonsmokers.[33] Nonetheless, the executive function is the most affected cognitive domain possibly because of vascular pathways involvement in this domain.[34]

To note, people with dementia are thought to have low rates of smoking; however, the main reason is not clear.[35]

Effect on mental health

Smoking might modulate the activity of some psychotropic medications. It induces cytochrome P450, mainly the CYP1A2, thus, interfering with the metabolism of antipsychotics like clozapine and olanzapine. A study showed that the plasma concentration of clozapine in smokers is 81.8% of that of nonsmokers.[36] Smokers experience less sedation and drowsiness with certain benzodiazepines, mainly diazepam and chlordiazepoxide.[24]

In addition, smokers have a high level of CYP2B6, the enzyme responsible for serotonin and testosterone metabolism, as well as nicotine, cocaine, amphetamines, and bupropion.[37]

Some hypothesized that smoking may be incriminated in the onset and maintenance of anxiety and bipolar disorders.[23]

In addition, people with psychiatric disorders are at double the risk of smoking and have 25% less chance of quitting smoking.[38,39]

Benefits of smoking

Smoking may provide some benefits in certain health conditions. In fact, it was found that smoking may delay and protect people from having ulcerative colitis; however, smoking cessation should be advocated in this population, knowing that it can cause many deadly smoking-related diseases.[40] Furthermore, smoking was found to have a positive effect on endometrial cancer[41] and Parkinson disease. In fact, there is a reduction in the prevalence of Parkinson disease between smokers and nonsmokers, and ex-smokers and nonsmokers. A study performed showed that the risk of Parkinson disease was 41% lower in smokers compared with nonsmokers.[42] Smoking is beneficial for Parkinson through several mechanisms. First, nicotine stimulates dopaminergic neurons in the brain, which relieves Parkinson disease symptoms and has a neuroprotective effect. Second, nicotine inactivates monoamine oxidase B enzyme, which is responsible for the activation of the parkinsonian-inducing neurotoxins.[31]

In addition, smoking has a positive effect on multiple cognitive domains. A meta-analysis done in 2010 shows a significant positive effect of nicotine on fine motor abilities, attention, and memory.[43]

Smoking Cessation

Counseling

Encouraging smoking cessation and promoting health should be a major part of the physician-patient encounter. It is very important for the patient to understand the disadvantages of smoking and their health-related consequences. A critical component is to educate the patient about the advantages and the benefits of smoking cessation at any age, especially in the elderly population. The topic of smoking cessation should be discussed during every patient-physician encounter even if the patient is not ready. The clinician should also motivate the patient by offering assistance, advice, and encouragement. The physician should reassure the patient that he will guide him through the process and offer him replacement therapies, group therapies, exercises, and time-management strategies to relieve the stressful period.[44,45]

According to the United States Prevention Services Task Force,[46] physicians should regularly ask about tobacco use and should encourage stopping. They recommend the 5 A's approach for counseling:

1. Ask about tobacco
2. Advise to quit
3. Assess willingness to quit
4. Assist in quitting
5. Arrange a follow-up and support

However, some investigators considered that smoking cessation might reduce the coping ability of the elderly and their quality of life; thus, the risk for stopping smoking might outweigh the benefits.[43]

Older adults exhibit low interest in attempting quitting because of their low ability to understand the harms and risk of smoking, notably among the cognitively impaired.[36]

Medical Therapy

Several pharmacologic therapies can help in smoking cessation.

Nicotine replacement therapy

Nicotine replacement therapy, such as lozenges, transdermal patches, sprays, and gums, can be used as first-line treatment. Many studies found the positive effect of replacement therapies, prescribed in optimal and effective dosages, with or without behavioral therapies on smoking cessation.[2]

Pharmacodynamics of nicotine do not differ between elderly and young; thus, dosage modification is not necessary, and nicotine therapy will not have an enhanced effect in the elderly. To note, nicotine is excreted through the kidneys, so cautious usage of replacement should be done in the case of renal impairment.[2]

Bupropion

Bupropion, an antidepressant, is effective for smoking cessation, alone or in combination with nicotine replacement therapy. It should be prescribed at a dose of 150 mg/d the first 3 days and then 150 mg twice daily for 8 to 10 weeks. Studies have shown noninferiority and sometimes superiority in the quitting rates between bupropion and replacement therapies. However, bupropion has many adverse effects, and the noncompliance rates are higher than in the nicotine replacement therapy.[2] Bupropion is contraindicated in those with seizures or a history of anorexia or bulimia. It can cause cognitive impairment and motor impairment, so it should be used cautiously in the elderly at the risk of delirium. It can cause weight loss that is detrimental in the elderly population and can be one of the main events promoting frailty. Furthermore, it can accumulate in the elderly because of chronic dosing, so low doses should be used in frail older people.[47]

Clonidine and nortriptyline

Clonidine and nortriptyline are considered second-line agents. Clonidine might decrease the craving for cigarettes.[2] It can be given either orally or transdermally. Studies have shown that the chances of quitting were increased by 90% with clonidine. However, it should be used cautiously in the elderly because it can cause hypotension, bradycardia, central nervous system depression, respiratory depression, and xerostomia.[48]

Nortriptyline was shown to double the quitting rates in 6 placebo-controlled trials. The doses used in trials were 75 mg to 100 mg. Data are lacking about the dose-dependent side effects in smokers, because small trials were performed. The fact that nortriptyline and bupropion help in smoking cessation, but not selective serotonin reuptake inhibitors, may be due to the important role of dopaminergic and noradrenergic but not serotonergic receptors in cessation.[49]

Although nortriptyline is a secondary amine, having the lowest side effects among other tricyclic antidepressants, it can cause anticholinergic side effects: xerostomia, constipation, blurry vision, urinary retention, and cognitive impairment. Previous studies have shown that 30% of patients over the age of 40 years develops delirium while being treated with tricyclics. Thus, it should be avoided in the elderly.[50]

Varenicline

Varenicline is an alpha4-beta2 neuronal nicotinic acetylcholine receptor partial agonist approved for smoking cessation. It is started at low doses and incrementally increased each 3 days to reach a 1-mg twice-daily dose after day 7, and this maintenance dose is taken over 11 weeks. The pharmacokinetics of this medication do not differ between gender, age, or ethnicities; however, it is renally cleared so it should be used cautiously in renal impairment.[51] This medication should be used cautiously, because it can cause a wide spectrum of neuropsychiatric effects, notably depression and suicidality.[52] In 1 retrospective study in older adults, patients who received varenicline were 3.22 times more likely to quit smoking than those who received Nicotine replacement therapy (NRT).[53]

Alternative Medicine Options

Some patients are referred to hypnosis or acupuncture as an alternative treatment to traditional medicine.[2] Cognitive behavioral therapy is also an important method for smoking cessation mainly in the elderly. Cognitive behavioral therapy can lead to high rates of stopping cigarettes and maintaining smoking cessation in both men and women.[54]

Electronic Cigarettes

Electronic cigarettes have recently been used as a means for smoking cessation (35.5% of adults and 25.3% in the last 3 months)[55] as a transitory phase. However, they can push people, especially the young generation, aged 18 to 24 (24.5%) and 25 to 44 years (49.3%),[56] to start tobacco products. Data from 2018 estimate that around 1% of persons aged more than 65 years old use e-cigarettes and vaping.[57] The long-term health effect of electronic cigarettes is currently unknown: they still contain tobacco, and they also burn chemicals.[58]

SUMMARY

In summary, nicotine use disorder is common among the elderly, and many succeed quitting smoking for personal reasons or for health-related issues. Smoking causes many health problems, attacking all the systems in the body and shortening lifespan. However, other people either fail to or refuse to quit smoking because of their possible poor knowledge and insight about its side effects, or because they find it a pleasure or a stress reliever. Therefore, an appropriate counseling and smoking cessation approach is required at every visit, and several methods of cessation can be proposed, from nicotine replacement to medications to alternative medicine. Anyone at any age can stop smoking! Age is not an excuse!

CLINICS CARE POINTS

- Smoking is a major risk factor for the development of chronic diseases, including cardiovascular, respiratory system, eyes, gums, and bones, that can have debilitating consequences on the elderly. It is also associated with increased risk of cancer.
- Smoking cessation in older adults should be prioritized. The primary care physician/geriatrician should assess and advise quitting at each encounter.
- Several treatment strategies pharmacologic and nonpharmacologic can be used and should be tailored for each patient while taking into account the adverse events and the comorbidities.

DISCLOSURE

The authors have nothing to disclose.

REFERENCES

1. Woods M. Smoking cessation for older adults: it's not too late! Beth Israel Lahey Health Winchester Hospital web site. Available at: https://www. winchesterhospital.org/health-library/article?id=13490. Accessed April 20, 2021.
2. Appel DW, Aldrich TK. Smoking cessation in the elderly. Clin Geriatr Med 2003; 19(1):77–100.
3. Tobacco- related disorders. In: American Psychiatric Association: desk reference to the diagnostic criteria from DSM-5. Arlington (VA): American Psychiatric association; 2013. p. 274–7.
4. Kleykamp BA, Heishman SJ. The older smoker. JAMA 2011;306(8):876–7.
5. Blazer DG, Wu L. Patterns of tobacco use and tobacco-related psychiatric morbidity and substance use among middle-aged and older adults in the United States. Aging Ment Health 2012;16(3):296–304.
6. Tobacco consumption statistics. Available at: https://ec.europa.eu/eurostat/ statistics-explained/index.php?title=Tobacco_consumption_statistics. Accessed April 20, 2021.
7. Ossip-Klein D, Pearson T, McIntosh S, et al. Smoking is a geriatric health issue. Nicotine Tob Res 1999;1(4):299–300.
8. Bjarnason NH, Mikkelsen KL, Tønnesen P. Smoking habits and beliefs about smoking in elderly patients with COPD during hospitalisation. J Smok Cessat 2010;5(1):15–21.
9. Degenhardt L, Hall W, Lynskey M. Alcohol, cannabis and tobacco use among Australians: a comparison of their associations with other drug use and use disorders, affective and anxiety disorders, and psychosis. Addiction 2001;96(11): 1603–14.
10. Glover-Bondeau A. Le tabagisme des seniors. 2019. Available at: https://www. stop-tabac.ch/fr/le-tabagisme-des-seniors. Accessed April 20, 2021.
11. Tobacco use. Available at: https://www.cdc.gov/chronicdisease/resources/ publications/factsheets/tobacco.htm. Accessed April 20, 2021.
12. Gellert C, Schöttker B, Brenner H. Smoking and all-cause mortality in older people: systematic review and meta-analysis. Arch Intern Med 2012;172(11):837–44.
13. Nadruz J, Wilson, Claggett B, Gonçalves A, et al. Smoking and cardiac structure and function in the elderly: the ARIC study. Circ Cardiovasc Imaging 2016;9(9): e004950.
14. Pan B, Jin X, Jun L, et al. The relationship between smoking and stroke. Medicine (Baltimore) 2019;98(12):e14872.
15. Smoking and cardiovascular disease. Available at: https://www.cdc.gov/tobacco/ data_statistics/sgr/50th-anniversary/pdfs/fs_smoking_CVD_508.pdf. Accessed April 20, 2021.
16. Pittilo M. Cigarette smoking, endothelial injury and cardiovascular disease. Int J Exp Pathol 2000;81(4):219–30.
17. Ambrose JA, Barua RS. The pathophysiology of cigarette smoking and cardiovascular disease. J Am Coll Cardiol 2004;43(10):1731–7.
18. Atkinson J. COPD: pathogenesis, epidemiology, and the role of cigarette smoke. Pulmonary Advisor Web site Available at: https://www.pulmonologyadvisor.-com>home>copd. Updated 2017. Accessed April 20, 2021.
19. Reh DD, Higgins TS, Smith TL. Impact of tobacco smoke on chronic rhinosinusitis: a review of the literature. Int Forum Allergy Rhinol 2012;2(5):362–9.
20. Reh D, Higgins T, Smith T. Impact of tobacco smoke on chronic rhinosinusitis – a review of the literature. Int Forum Allergy Rhinol 2012;2(5):362–9.

21. What are the risk factors for lung cancer?. Available at: https://www.cdc.gov/cancer/lung/basic_info/risk_factors.htm. Accessed April 20, 2021.

22. Hernlgou J, Schulnd F. Tobacco and bone fractures. Bone Jt Res 2019;8:255–65.

23. Raju P, George R, Ramesh SV, et al. Influence of tobacco use on cataract development. Br J Ophthalmol 2006;90(11):1374–7.

24. Velilla S, García-Medina JJ, García-Layana A, et al. Smoking and age-related macular degeneration: review and update. J Ophthalmol 2013;2013:895147.

25. Leung WC, Harvey I. Epidemiology and health service research: is skin ageing in the elderly caused by sun exposure or smoking. Br J Dermatol 2002;147:1187–91.

26. Benowitz NL. Pharmacology of nicotine: addiction, smoking-induced disease, and therapeutics. Annu Rev Pharmacol Toxicol 2009;49(1):57–71.

27. Almeida O, Garrido G, Lautenschlager N, et al. Smoking is associated with reduced cortical regional gray matter density in brain regions associated with incipient Alzheimer disease. Am J Geriatr Psychiatry 2008;16(1):92–8.

28. Swan GE, Lessov-Schlaggar CN. The effects of tobacco smoke and nicotine on cognition and the brain. Neuropsychol Rev 2007;17:259–73.

29. Sabia S, Elbaz A, Dugravot A, et al. Impact of smoking on cognitive decline in early old age: the Whitehall II cohort study. Arch Gen Psychiatry 2012;69(6):627–35.

30. Cataldo JK, Prochaska JJ, Glantz SA. Cigarette smoking is a risk factor for Alzheimer's disease: an analysis controlling for tobacco industry affiliation. J Alzheimers Dis 2010;19(2):465–80.

31. Cataldo JK, Glantz SA. Smoking cessation and Alzheimer's disease: facts, fallacies and promise. Expert Rev Neurother 2010;10(5):629–31.

32. Livingston G, Sommerlad A, Orgeta V, et al. Dementia prevention, intervention, and care. Lancet 2017;390(10113):2673–734.

33. Nooyens AC, van Gelder BM, Verschuren WM. Smoking and cognitive decline among middle-aged men and women: the Doetinchem cohort study. Am J Public Health 2008;98(12):2244–50.

34. Peters R, Poulter R, Warner J, et al. Smoking, dementia and cognitive decline in the elderly, a systematic review. BMC Geriatr 2008;8(1):36.

35. Lester PE, Lyubarova R, Kirtani V, et al. Smoking rates in dementia patients in the outpatient setting. Arch Gerontol Geriatr 2010;52(3):281–3.

36. Zevin S, Benowitz NL. Drug interactions with tobacco smoking. Clin Pharmacokinet 1999;36(6):425–38.

37. Boksa P, PhD. Smoking, psychiatric illness and the brain. J Psychiatry Neurosci 2017;42(3):147–9.

38. Asharani PV, Ling Seet VA, Abdin E, et al. Smoking and mental illness: prevalence, patterns and correlates of smoking and smoking cessation among psychiatric patients. Int J Environ Res Public Health 2020;17(15):5571.

39. Sachs-Ericsson N, Collins N, Schmidt B, et al. Older adults and smoking: characteristics, nicotine dependence and prevalence of DSM-IV 12-month disorders. Aging Ment Health 2011;15(1):132–41.

40. To N, Ford AC, Gracie DJ. Systematic review with meta-analysis: the effect of tobacco smoking on the natural history of ulcerative colitis. Aliment Pharmacol Ther 2016;44(2):117.

41. Terry PD, Rohan TE, Franceschi S, et al. Smoking and endometrial cancer cigarette smoking and the risk of endometrial cancer. Lancet Oncol 2002;3(8):470–80.

42. Li X, Li W, Liu G, et al. Association between cigarette smoking and Parkinson's disease: a meta-analysis. Am J Geriatr Psychiatry 2015;61(3):510–6.
43. Heishman S, Kleykamp B, Singleton E. Meta-analysis of the acute effects of nicotine and smoking on human performance. Psychopharmacology 2010;210(4): 453–69.
44. Chen D, Wu L. Smoking cessation interventions for adults aged 50 or older: a systematic review and meta-analysis. Drug Alcohol Depend 2015;154:14–24.
45. Lande G. Nicotine addiction treatment & management. Medscape Web site. Available at: https://emedicine.medscape.com>287555-treatment. Updated 2018. Accessed April 25, 2021.
46. Krist AH, Davidson KW, Mangione CM, et al. Interventions for tobacco smoking cessation in adults, including pregnant persons: US Preventive Services Task Force recommendation statement. JAMA 2021;325(3):265–79.
47. Clinical Practice Guideline Treating Tobacco Use and Dependence 2008 Update Panel, Liaisons, and Staff. A clinical practice guidelines for treating tobacco use and dependence: 2008 update. A U.S. public health service report. Am J Prev Med 2008;35(2):158–76.
48. Cahill k, Stevens S, Perera R, et al. Pharmacological interventions for smoking cessation: an overview and network meta-analysis. Cochrane Database Syst Rev 2013;(5):CD009329.
49. Hughes J, Stead L, Lancaster T. Nortriptyline for smoking cessation: a review. Nicotine Tob Res 2005;7(4):491–9.
50. Mccue RE. Using tricyclic antidepressants in the elderly. Clin Geriatr Med 1992; 8(2):323–34.
51. Ravva P, Gastonguay MR, Tensfeldt TG, et al. Population pharmacokinetic analysis of varenicline in adult smokers. Br J Clin Pharmacol 2009;68(5):669–81.
52. Anthenelli RM, Benowitz NL, West R, et al. Neuropsychiatric safety and efficacy of varenicline, bupropion, and nicotine patch in smokers with and without psychiatric disorders (EAGLES): a double-blind, randomised, placebo-controlled clinical trial. Lancet 2016;387(10037):2507–20.
53. Chang CP, Huang WH, You CH, et al. Factors correlated with smoking cessation success in older adults: a retrospective cohort study in Taiwan. Int J Environ Res Public Health 2019;16(18):3462.
54. Hall SM, Humfleet GL, Muñoz RF, et al. Extended treatment of older cigarette smokers. Addiction 2009;104(6):1043–52.
55. Carabello R, Shafer P, Patel D, et al. Quit methods used by US adult cigarette smokers, 2014-216. Prev Chronic Dis 2017;14:E32.
56. Cornelius ME, Wang TW, Jamal A, et al. Tobacco product use among adults United States, 2019. MMWR Morb Mortal Wkly Rep 2020;69(46):1736–42.
57. Bao W, Liu B, Du Y, et al. Electronic cigarette use among young, middle-aged, and older adults in the United States in 2017 and 2018. JAMA Intern Med 2020;180(2):313–4.
58. United States Public Health Service Office of the Surgeon General, National Center for Chronic Disease Prevention and Health Promotion (US) Office on Smoking and Health. Smoking cessation: a report of the surgeon general. Washington (DC): US Department of Health and Human Services; 2020.

A Brewed Awakening
Neuropsychiatric Effects of Caffeine in Older Adults

Ellen Kim, MD, Neil M. Robinson, Brianne M. Newman, MD*

KEYWORDS

- Caffeine • Older adults • Cognition • Late-life depression • Insomnia

KEY POINTS

- Daily caffeine consumption is common among older adults in the United States, although prevalence data on caffeine use disorder in this population is lacking.
- Although multiple studies have shown caffeine use may be related to decreased risk of Alzheimer's disease, research demonstrates conflicting associations between caffeine, cognitive disorders and benefits on cognition.
- Long-term caffeine intake is inversely associated with the risk of developing Parkinson's disease. However, the potential of caffeine to alleviate the motor symptoms of parkinsonism may be temporary, if at all.
- Regular caffeine consumption has demonstrated possible protective effects against the development of late-life depression via a decrease in neuroinflammation. However, artificial sweeteners often used in caffeinated beverages may increase the risk of depression.
- In older adults, anxiety often goes underdiagnosed and undertreated. Caffeine is a well-known anxiogenic agent and high caffeine consumption can exacerbate generalized anxiety disorders in older adults.
- Caffeine can have psychopharmacological interactions with drugs metabolized in the liver by the CYP450 system, such as fluvoxamine, clozapine, zolpidem, whereas caffeine withdrawal may impact renal clearance of lithium.

CAFFEINE USE, DEPENDENCE, AND USE DISORDER

Caffeine is the most consumed drug in the United States, with more than 85% of adults regularly ingesting caffeine at average doses of more than 200 mg/d (>2 cups of coffee or 5 cans of soda).[1,2] The extensive nonproblematic use of caffeine in the general population, as well as the possible health benefits of mild to moderate caffeine intake, make the line between use and misuse unclear. Similarly,

Department of Psychiatry & Behavioral Neuroscience, Saint Louis University School of Medicine, 1438 Grand Boulevard, Saint Louis, MO 63104, USA
* Corresponding author.
E-mail address: brianne.newman@health.slu.edu

Clin Geriatr Med 38 (2022) 133–144
https://doi.org/10.1016/j.cger.2021.07.009
0749-0690/22/© 2021 Elsevier Inc. All rights reserved.

psychological and physiological reactions to the same amount of caffeine can vary owing to individual factors such as hepatic enzyme function, age, lean body mass, and other genetic factors.[2,3] A recent epidemiologic study found that 86.4% of adults age 60 or older report caffeine consumption in the form of coffee, with 69.2% of older adults reporting daily coffee consumption.[4] Another population-based study of elderly patients in Spain showed significantly increased coffee use in older adults age 75 or older ($P = .02$), with smoking tobacco and drinking alcohol as the 2 main factors associated with greater consumption.[5]

Published studies often term caffeine dependence as an individual's inability to control caffeine use despite negative physical or psychological consequences associated with continued use.[2] Diagnostic criteria for both caffeine intoxication and caffeine withdrawal are considered well-validated diagnostic entities and are listed in the fifth edition of the *Diagnostic and Statistical Manual of Mental Disorders* (DSM-5) section on substance-related and addictive disorders. Advancing age is noted as a possible contributor to more severe physiological reaction to caffeine, possibly increasing risk for caffeine intoxication.[6] The World Health Organization developed *The International Statistical Classification of Diseases and Related Health Problems*, which also identifies a specific diagnosis, caffeine use syndrome, for problematic caffeine use causing functional impairment.[7,8]

Caffeine use disorder first appeared in the DSM-5 in 2013, as a condition for further study.[6] Despite the known biological possibility of an individual developing problematic substance use disorder with caffeine, there has been concern about overpathologizing habitual but nonproblematic caffeine use. Budney and colleagues[6] discuss the validity concerns with caffeine use disorder,[9] highlighting the diagnostic specifics in the DSM-5 that attempt to address overdiagnosis. Unlike the other substance use disorders, caffeine use disorder requires 3 key criteria (repeated unsuccessful attempts to quit or cut down, withdrawal, and continued use despite harm).[6] It also includes the same criteria for causing clinically significant distress or impairment in functioning as the other substance use disorders in an attempt to limit the overpathologizing of nonproblematic caffeine use.

Specific data on the prevalence of caffeine use disorder in older adults is sparse. Changes in diagnostic criteria limit consistent data. Meredith and colleagues reviewed existing epidemiologic prevalence data using the DSM-5 criteria and reported an approximate 9% prevalence rate for caffeine use disorder in the general population.[2] Although this study did provide data on a few subpopulations, specific data for the elderly were not reported. Sweeney and colleagues[10] published a very recent general population study in the United States focused caffeine use disorder based on DSM-5 criteria. Similar to Meredith and colleagues' findings,[2] this study reported a general population prevalence of 8% meeting the core 3 criteria for caffeine use disorder.[10] The authors note that the average age was 47.4 ± 16.4 years, but women, smokers, and older adults were over-represented in the sample compared with the general US population.[10]

CAFFEINE PHARMACOLOGY

Caffeine is often consumed for its psychostimulant properties, such as improved alertness, energy, and mood. Caffeine is absorbed in the gastrointestinal tract and can cross the blood–brain barrier, with peak plasma concentrations after oral absorption in 15 to 120 minutes. It is metabolized by the liver cytochrome P450 system (CYP), with the cytochrome P450 1A2 (*CYP1A2*) enzyme playing an important role in the metabolism of caffeine. Thus, genetic polymorphisms in the *CYP1A2* gene or hepatic dysfunction can affect caffeine metabolism and have been associated with individual caffeine intake.[2,11]

Caffeine is a potent inhibitor of adenosine receptors, specifically A_1 and A_{2A}. A_{2A} adenosine receptors are most heavily concentrated in the dopaminergic areas of the brain. Changes in dopaminergic activity in areas such as the nucleus accumbens may be related to the development of dependence in some individuals.[2,11] Genetic variations in adenosine receptors may contribute to individual differences in caffeine's effect on sleep, anxiety, and physiological response.

CAFFEINE AND COGNITION

Caffeine's effect on cognition has been examined in observational studies and animal models. Although acute intake of caffeine reveals cognitive benefits, studies investigating the effects of long-term intake on cognitive function yield unclear results.

Recently, 2 cross-sectional analyses evaluated data from the National Health and Nutritional Examination Surveys (NHANES) to assess the effect of caffeine consumption on cognitive domains (executive function, memory, and attention) among US adults ages 60 years or older.[12,13] Validated measurements included the Consortium to Establish a Registry for Alzheimer's disease (CERAD) Word Recall test, which is part of a validated instrument to assess for Alzheimer's disease (AD), and the Digit Symbol Substitution Test, which tests for motor speech, attention, and visuoperceptual functions. The first analysis included NHANES 2013 to 2014 data and accounted for all caffeine-containing sources.[12] Results showed, after adjusting for confounders (eg, age, sex, medical comorbidities), that there was a borderline nonsignificant association in the CERAD World List Recall test ($P = .09$) and the highest quartile of caffeine intake (170.9 ± 11.8 mg), but not in other cognitive domains.[12] The second analysis included NHANES 2011 to 2012 and 2013 to 2014 data, and only accounted for caffeine from coffee. Results showed those who reported use of 266.4 to 495.0 mg of coffee per day had significantly higher Digit Symbol Substitution Test and CERAD test scores, with the association more significant in women.[13] Given these results, the impact of caffeine or other components of coffee on cognition remains unclear.

A Mendelian randomization meta-analysis of 415,540 European participants examined the causal relationship between habitual coffee intake and cognitive function in mid- to later-life.[14] The study chose 2 common genetic variants that had the strongest biological influence on habitual caffeine intake, the *CYP1A1/2* and the aryl-hydrocarbon receptor genes. Results showed a null association between the long-term effects of coffee intake on global cognition and memory. Another study investigated the effect of coffee on brain MRI markers of dementia and cognitive performance measurements.[15] Greater coffee consumption was associated with a lesser prevalence of lacunar infarcts and better executive function, but smaller hippocampal volume and worse memory function.

These inconsistent findings may be partially explained by methodological problems from studying dietary exposures, such as confounding and reverse causation, as well as variations in caffeine metabolism.[14] Additionally, major sources of caffeine, such as coffee and tea, have other substances (eg, theanine) that may affect cognition.[14]

CAFFEINE AND ALZHEIMER'S DISEASE

AD is the most common type of dementia, accounting for approximately 50% to 70% of dementia cases.[16] AD is a slowly progressive disease, characterized by early symptoms of short-term memory loss, apathy, and depression. The hallmark pathologic features are the accumulation of amyloid-β plaques in the gray matter of the brain and neurofibrillary tangles of protein tau inside neurons.[16]

Given the limited pharmacologic options for treating AD, there have been promising experimental studies on dietary interventions, such as caffeine use.[16] Animal studies suggest that caffeine has neuroprotective effects via amyloid-β–related pathways.[16] Caffeine acts as a nonselective adenosine A_1 and A_{2A} receptor antagonist. Blocking adenosine A_{2A} receptor has demonstrated attenuating amyloid-β–induced cognitive deficits in AD-transgenic mice.[16] However, clinical and epidemiologic studies testing this hypothesis have had equivocal results.

Positive studies between coffee consumption and cognitive disorders show a dose-response J-shaped curve relationship. A meta-analysis of 9 prospective cohort studies revealed that drinking 1 to 2 cups of coffee a day was inversely associated with cognitive disorders, but intake or more than 3 cups a day had nonsignificant cognitive impact.[17]

A recent cross-sectional study may provide a neuropathological reason for the positive association between coffee intake and reduced risk of AD. This study examined whether coffee decreases brain pathologic hallmarks of AD, including cerebral beta-amyloid deposition and cerebral white matter hyperintensities.[18] The participants were either cognitively normal adults or adults with mild cognitive impairment (n = 411; range, 55–90 years old). Exclusion criteria included drinking tea regularly. After controlling for confounders, results showed a lifetime coffee intake of 2 or more cups a day was significantly associated with lower cerebral beta-amyloid deposition positivity (27.14%) compared with coffee intake of less than 2 cups a day (17.61%). Furthermore, the relationship was more prominent for lifetime coffee intake than current coffee intake ($P = .003$ vs $P = .013$). However, these findings were not found with other markers of regional neurodegeneration and white matter hyperintensities. These results suggest that a greater lifetime coffee intake contributes to a lesser risk of AD or related cognitive decline by decreasing pathologic cerebral amyloid deposition.[18]

However, other studies have shown null associations. The Canadian Study of Health and Aging, a prospective cohort study, followed 6434 participants (ages ≥65 years) with normal cognition.[19] At the 5-year follow-up, daily consumption of coffee decreased the risk of AD by 31%. However, when including participants who died during the 5-year follow-up period, the protective effect of coffee consumption was not statistically significant.[19] A recent meta-analysis of 8 prospective studies concluded that no statistically significant relationship between coffee consumption and risk of dementia, with similar findings in a subgroup meta-analysis of the studies specifically on AD.[20]

CAFFEINE AND PARKINSON'S DISEASE

Parkinson's disease (PD) is a neurodegenerative disease that involves the progressive depletion of dopaminergic neurons in the basal ganglia, particularly the substantia nigra. It is the second most common neurodegenerative disease and characterized by motor and nonmotor symptoms.[21]

Several large epidemiologic studies have demonstrated neuroprotective effects of caffeine on PD. The neuroprotective effects are hypothesized to involve adenosine A_{2A} receptor antagonism, which downregulates the phosphatidylinositol 3-kinase/protein kinase B signaling pathways and prevents excessive calcium release, which is associated with neurotoxicity and neuroinflammation.[21]

The Honolulu Heart Program, a prospective longitudinal study, followed 8004 Japanese-American men (range, 45–68 years old) for 30 years.[22] The study demonstrated that, after adjusting for age and smoking status, the incidence of PD decreased by more than 5-fold for those who drank at least 28 oz of coffee a day compared with those who did not drink coffee.[22] A similar finding was observed with caffeine from noncoffee sources. A meta-analysis of 13 articles showed a dose–response relationship, with the maximum strength of protection at 3 cups of coffee a day (n = 901,764).[23] Gender differences may also play a role in the risk of developing PD, specifically owing to the interaction of caffeine and estrogen. Caffeine intake was associated with decreased risk of PD in postmenopausal women who did not use hormone replacement therapy, but not among women and postmenopausal women who had used hormone replacement therapy.[24]

Although studies have linked caffeine to a lower risk of PD, the effects of caffeine on symptoms of PD, specifically the motor benefits, have not shown similar results. Based on positive findings from a few small studies,[25,26] caffeine was further investigated in a multicenter, parallel-group controlled trial in patients who had PD from 1 to 8 years on stable managed therapy, with primary outcomes of motor score improvement in 6 months (n = 121).[27] Exclusion criteria included caffeine intake of more than 150 mg/d. Although caffeine was well-tolerated, there was no improvement in motor parkinsonism with caffeine 200 mg twice daily compared with placebo at 6 months of follow-up.[27] Additionally, on secondary outcomes, there was a small increase in dyskinesia with caffeine and a decrease in cognitive testing scores.[27] Given the longer trial length, caffeine may have short-term protective effects that wane with prolonged exposure. The increased dyskinesia may be attributed to exposure time. For example, caffeine may prevent dyskinesia if provided before dopamine therapy, but increase it if provided after.[27]

CAFFEINE AND INSOMNIA

Insomnia disorder manifests as dissatisfaction with sleep owing to difficulty initiating sleep, maintaining sleep, or awakening early in the morning.[6] Insomnia is prevalent among older adults. A recent study found that more than 70% of adults aged 65 and older report at least 1 symptom of insomnia.[28] In a systematic review of studies conducted in the general population, caffeine use negatively affected both objective and perceived sleep quality, causing increased sleep latency, and decreased sleep time and efficiency.[29] Late-life insomnia has been associated with significant cardiovascular and psychiatric comorbidities, with evidence strongly supporting insomnia and daytime sleepiness as independent risk factors for depression in older adults.[30,31] Therefore, understanding the relationship of caffeine consumption and insomnia in the aging population is clinically significant.

A recent cross-sectional survey study in Brazil examined the relationship of caffeine-induced insomnia with age and sex in a general population of adults aged 18 to 75 years.[32] Insomnia attributed to caffeine intake was found to increase with age in both male and female participants, even when adjusting for covariates such as sociodemographic characteristics, psychiatric comorbidities, and other sleep-related variables.[32] Older individuals who reported insomnia owing to caffeine use were more likely to use hypnotic drugs on a daily basis and had a greater prevalence of psychiatric diagnoses compared with their counterparts without caffeine-induced insomnia.[32] A cross-sectional survey study of adults aged 60 and older in Pakistan showed that patients who consumed caffeine within 2 hours before going to bed had an adjusted odds ratio of 6.5 for insomnia.[33]

Another study assessed the within-subject effects of caffeine use on sleep duration in middle-aged and older US adults aged 35 to 85 years using actinography, daily self-reported caffeine intake, and sleep logs.[34] Results demonstrated that older adults aged 55 to 85 years typically did not compensate for sleep loss with caffeine, compared with adults aged 35 to 55 years who tended to consume more caffeine to offset short sleep duration on prior nights.[34] Interestingly, this study found no association between daily caffeine use and sleep quantity, suggesting that regular caffeine consumption may not greatly impact sleep duration as the body becomes accustomed to habitual use.[34] This finding may be especially true in older adults, who tend to consume caffeine in the morning rather than throughout the day.[34,35]

Of note, the consumption of caffeine in adults older than 60 years has been shown to be associated with decreased levels of proinflammatory cytokine markers in individuals who sleep well at night compared with elevated cytokine levels in those with insomnia, indicating that, when tolerated, moderate caffeine intake may contribute to longevity by decreasing chronic inflammation.[36] Although coffee and tea both contain many bioactive compounds, research has shown that caffeine itself inhibits production of IL-1β, an important proinflammatory regulator; therefore, caffeine consumption may limit the effects of the inflammatory response caused by accumulation of harmful chemical byproducts as metabolic processes slow in older adults.[37] As a general guideline for older patients who wish to consume caffeinated products, a prior study showed that consumption of 400 mg of caffeine in middle-aged adults caused greater sleep disruptions than in younger adults, whereas both groups had less sleep sensitivity at a lower daily dose of 200 mg.[38]

CAFFEINE, DEPRESSION, AND ANXIETY

Depression in older adults is an important public health issue that has increasingly garnered attention as the number of older adults in aging populations increases worldwide.[39] Late-life depression is associated with disproportionately high rates of suicide as well as significant nonsuicide medical mortality.[36] Depression is related to many lifestyle factors, such as physical activity, alcohol consumption, nicotine intake, and dietary behaviors, including the consumption of caffeinated beverages.[40] A meta-analysis of observational studies in adults of all ages demonstrated that caffeine consumption is significantly associated with decreased risk of depression in the general population, with a dose-dependent response.[40] Recognizing the effects of caffeine on depression in older adults may help to discern its possible protective properties within this population.

Anxiety disorders often co-occur with depressive disorders.[41] Although more common than depressive disorders and found in 8% of older adults, anxiety disorders are often underdiagnosed.[41,42] Older adults are less likely to identify anxiety symptoms than younger adults and seek treatment.[41,43] Comorbid medical illnesses also confound presentations, making it easier for this diagnosis to be missed. Although most anxiety disorders in older adults begin at a younger age, about one-half of the cases of generalized anxiety disorder begin after the age of 50.[41] There are unique presentations of anxiety in older adults, such as a fear of falling, even for those without a history of falls and anxiety in patients with neurocognitive disorders.[42] Caffeine at high doses exacerbates underlying anxiety. Therefore, it is important to screen for all medications, dietary agents, and supplements. Scales specific to anxiety in older adults have shown to be more sensitive and accurate diagnostic tools than those for younger adults.[41]

In a cross-sectional study of Chinese adults aged 60 years and older, habitual tea drinkers were found to have better health-related quality of life as well as decreased rates of anxiety and depression, particularly with consumption of black or oolong tea.[44] Likewise, a cross-sectional study of rural-dwelling Chinese adults aged 60 years

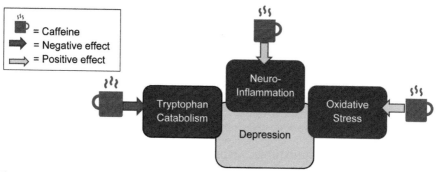

Figure 1. Relationship between caffeine and depression based on the neuroinflammatory hypothesis. (*Adapted from* Hall S, Desbrow B, Anoopkumar-Dukie S, et al. A review of the bioactivity of coffee, caffeine and key coffee constituents on inflammatory responses linked to depression. Food Res Int. 2015;76(3):628; with permission.)

and older showed a linear association of tea consumption with a decreased likelihood of depressive symptoms, demonstrating a statistically nonsignificant odds ratio of 0.86 with weekly intake and a significant odds ratio of 0.59 with daily intake.[45] An analysis of data from the Korean National Health and Nutrition Examination Survey found that after adjusting for confounding variables, the prevalence of self-reported lifetime depression was 21% lower in individuals who consumed at least 3 cups of green tea per week compared with those who did not drink tea.[46] Furthermore, those who drank 2 or more cups of coffee per day had a 32% lower prevalence of lifetime depression compared with those who did not drink coffee.[46] Similar findings that greater caffeine intake (median 284.9 mg; range, 234.9–758.0 mg) correlates with a decreased prevalence of depressive symptoms was found in a multicenter cross-sectional study of Japanese women aged 65 to 94 years, though the association was specific to coffee (median, 194 mg; range, 107–619 mg), rather than other caffeinated beverages.[47]

Studies conducted in US populations of older adults have demonstrated similar findings to the international literature. An analysis of a large dataset from NHANES found that regular caffeine intake had a stronger negative correlation with depressive symptoms in adults 70 years and older compared with younger age groups; each 1-mg increase in daily caffeine intake was associated with a multivariate beta value of −0.002 for depressive symptoms in adults 70 years and older, compared with −0.001 in individuals 45 to 69 years old and 0.001 in those 18 to 44 years old.[48] In a 10-year prospective study of a female cohort with a mean age of 63 years at study onset, the multivariate relative risk of depression was found to be 0.85 in women who drank 2 to 3 cups of coffee per day and 0.80 in those who drank 4 or more cups per day when compared with individuals who drank less than 1 cup per week.[49] Another prospective study in older, retired US adults also showed that frequent coffee consumption (>2 cups; $P = .0026$ for trend) was associated with a decreased risk of subsequent development of depression compared with nondrinkers; however, intake of diet soda and the addition of artificial sweeteners to coffee or tea was associated with increased risk of depression.[50]

Coffee contains multiple bioactive compounds, including caffeine, chlorogenic acid, ferulic acid, and caffeic acid, which have all been shown to decrease neuroinflammation and oxidative stress in the brain in both in vitro and in vivo studies.[51] Considering that neuroinflammation may be linked to depression pathophysiology, the anti-inflammatory properties of these compounds could explain the beneficial effects of coffee consumption in reducing depressive symptoms and behaviors.[51] The relationship between depression and the bioactive compounds found in coffee is further explored in **Fig. 1**. Conversely, the breakdown products of aspartame, a popular artificial sweetener often used in coffee and tea, are thought to cause decreased levels of serotonin and dopamine in the brain owing to elevated phenylalanine activity, and can also lead to the degeneration of neurons through aspartic acid–mediated excitotoxicity.[52] Overall, these findings suggest that regular, moderate consumption of caffeine in the form of coffee or tea may provide protective benefits against late-life depression, although patients should be wary when opting for beverages with artificial sweeteners.

INTERACTIONS WITH PSYCHOTROPIC MEDICATIONS

Although in healthy adults the half-life of caffeine is between 3 and 7 hours, it may take 33% longer to metabolize caffeine in older adults.[53] Therefore, older adults may be more susceptible to interactions between caffeine and psychotropic medications. Several clinically relevant interactions are summarized; additional interactions are included in **Table 1**.

Fluvoxamine, a selective serotonin reuptake inhibitor, is a potent inhibitor of *CYP1A2* and has led to increased plasma concentrations of caffeine. Studies in healthy volunteers have found that fluvoxamine decreased elimination of caffeine by up to 80% and increased the half-life of caffeine by 500%.[54] Fluvoxamine coadministered with caffeine can lead to the accumulation of caffeine to an extent that restriction of the latter may be warranted.[54]

Clozapine, an atypical antipsychotic often used for treatment-resistant schizophrenia, is extensively metabolized by *CYP1A2*.[55] Clozapine has a higher affinity than caffeine for the *CYP1A2* enzyme. However, because of the greater caffeine concentrations, caffeine likely occupies most of the *CYP1A2* binding sites, which inhibits clozapine metabolism and increases its concentration, leading to an increased risk of adverse events, such as agranulocytosis and seizures.[55]

Caffeine withdrawal has been hypothesized to increase lithium concentration owing to decreased renal lithium clearance.[56] Two case reports described patients who developed worsening lithium-associated tremor after the elimination of caffeine intake.[56] Another prospective, nonblinded study showed that patients managed stably on lithium had significantly increased serum lithium concentrations after withdrawal of caffeine from diet.[56]

Zolpidem, a short-acting hypnotic, is a gamma-aminobutyric acid benzodiazepine agonist that is partially metabolized by *CYP1A2*. Caffeine has been shown to mildly enhance zolpidem sedation.[57] This paradoxic effect is hypothesized to occur because caffeine reduces the pool of reactive oxygen species.[57] This process is theorized to increase the availability of melatonin to interact with zolpidem. This potential side effect of caffeine points to a need for further research on antioxidants potentially aiding in sleep.[57]

SUMMARY

There is a correlation between caffeine use and various neuropsychiatric disorders, with caffeine consumed at approximately 200 to 300 mg/d (equivalent to 2–3 cups of coffee) demonstrating protective benefits. This review highlights the need for studies that clarify the impact of caffeine or a combination of caffeine with other biologically active ingredients in major sources of caffeine (coffee, tea, and soda) on neuropsychiatric disorders. There is also a need for high-quality randomized controlled trials and prospective studies to assess the potential benefits of caffeine. In the area of cognition,

Table 1
Psychopharmacologic medications that affect caffeine pharmacokinetics

Class	Name	Interaction with Caffeine
Serotonin norepinephrine reuptake inhibitor	Venlafaxine	No significant interaction
Selective serotonin reuptake inhibitor	Fluvoxamine	Decreases caffeine $t_{1/2}$ down to 80%
Tricyclic antidepressant	Clomipramine	May increase caffeine $t_{1/2}$
	Desipramine	May increase caffeine $t_{1/2}$
Atypical antipsychotic	Clozapine	Increases caffeine $t_{1/2}$ up to 25%
	Olanzapine	Mixed results, may decrease caffeine $t_{1/2}$
Benzodiazepine	Alprazolam	No significant effect
Mood stabilizer	Lithium	Caffeine decreases lithium concentrations through renal clearance
	Valproic acid	No significant interaction
	Carbamazepine	Caffeine prolong carbamazepine $t_{1/2}$
Nonbenzodiazepine hypnotic	Zolpidem	Mixed results, caffeine may decrease clearance of zolpidem

$t_{1/2}$, half-life.

Adapted from Carrillo JA, Benitez J. Clinically Significant Pharmacokinetic Interactions Between Dietary Caffeine and Medications. Clin Pharmacokinet. 2000;39(2):127-153; and Broderick PJ, Benjamin AB, Dennis LW. Caffeine and psychiatric medication interactions: a review. J Okla State Med Assoc. 2005;98(8):380-384; with permission.

whereas it is unclear if caffeine definitively impacts overall cognition, future studies should evaluate specific cognitive domains. Additionally, high consumption of caffeine can increase anxiety disorders, which is often undetected and undertreated in older adults. Future research should further explore this relationship in older adults. Finally, given caffeine's pharmacology, interactions with drugs, and the unique physiological changes with aging, it is important to recognize that the number of older adults who consume caffeine is high and caffeine use should be screened.

DISCLOSURE

The authors have nothing to disclose.

REFERENCES

1. Frary CD, Johnson RK, Wang MQ. Food sources and intakes of caffeine in the diets of persons in the United States. J Am Diet Assoc 2005;105:110–3.

2. Meredith SE, Juliano LM, Hughes JR, et al. Caffeine use disorder: a comprehensive review and research agenda. J Caffeine Res 2013;3(3):114–30.

3. Massey LK. Caffeine and the elderly. Drugs Aging 1998;13:43–50.

4. Loftfield E, Freedman ND, Dodd KW, et al. Coffee drinking is widespread in the United States, but usual intake varies by key demographic and lifestyle factors. J Nutr 2016;146(9):1762–8.

5. Torres-Collado L, García-de la Hera M, Navarrete-Muñoz EM, et al. Coffee drinking and associated factors in an elderly population in Spain. Int J Environ Res Public Health 2018;15(8):1661.

6. American Psychiatric Association. Diagnostic and statistical manual of mental disorders. 5th edition. Arlington: American Psychiatric Association; 2013.

7. World Health Organization. International statistical Classification of diseases and related health problems, 10th revision. Geneva (Switzerland): World Health Organization; 1992.

8. World Health Organization. The ICD-10 Classification of mental and behavioural disorders: clinical Descriptions and diagnostic guidelines. Geneva (Switzerland): World Health Organization; 1992.

9. Budney AJ, Lee DC, Juliano LM. Evaluating the validity of caffeine use disorder. Curr Psychiatry Rep 2015;17:74.

10. Sweeney MM, Weaver DC, Vincent KB, et al. Prevalence and correlates of caffeine use disorder symptoms among a United States sample. J Caffeine Adenosine Res 2020;10(1):4–11.

11. Fredholm BB, Battig K, Holmen J, v. Actions of caffeine in the brain with special reference to factors that contribute to its widespread use. Pharmacol Rev 1999; 51:83–133.

12. Iranpour S, Saadati HM, Koohi F, et al. Association between caffeine intake and cognitive function in adults; effect modification by sex: data from National Health and Nutrition Examination Survey (NHANES) 2013–2014. Clin Nutr 2020;39(7): 2158–68.

13. Dong X, Li S, Sun J, et al. Association of coffee, decaffeinated coffee and caffeine intake from coffee with cognitive performance in older adults: National Health and Nutrition Examination Survey (NHANES) 2011–2014. Nutrients 2020;12(3). https://doi.org/10.3390/nu12030840.

14. Zhou A, Taylor AE, Karhzunen V, et al. Habitual coffee consumption and cognitive function: a Mendelian randomization meta-analysis in up to 415,530 participants. Sci Rep 2018;8. https://doi.org/10.1038/s41598-018-25919-2.

15. Araújo LF, Giatti L, Reis RC, et al. Inconsistency of association between coffee consumption and cognitive function in adults and elderly in a cross-sectional study (ELSA-Brasil). Nutrients 2015;7(11):9590–601.

16. Londzin P, Zamora M, Kąkol B, et al. Potential of caffeine in Alzheimer's disease—a review of experimental studies. Nutrients 2021;13(2). https://doi.org/10.3390/nu13020537.

17. Wu L, Sun D, He Y. Coffee intake and the incident risk of cognitive disorders: a dose–response meta-analysis of nine prospective cohort studies. Clin Nutr 2017;36(3):730–6.

18. Kim JW, Byun MS, Yi D, et al. Coffee intake and decreased amyloid pathology in human brain. Translational Psychiatry 2019;9(1):1–10.

19. Lindsay J, Laurin D, Verreault R, et al. Risk factors for Alzheimer's disease: a prospective analysis from the Canadian study of health and aging. Am J Epidemiol 2002;156(5):445–53.

20. Larsson SC, Orsini N. Coffee consumption and risk of dementia and Alzheimer's disease: a dose-response meta-analysis of prospective studies. Nutrients 2018; 10(10). https://doi.org/10.3390/nu10101501.

21. Ascherio A, Schwarzschild MA. The epidemiology of Parkinson's disease: risk factors and prevention. Lancet Neurol 2016;15(12):1257–72.

22. Ross GW, Abbott RD, Petrovitch H, et al. Association of coffee and caffeine intake with the risk of Parkinson disease. JAMA 2000;283(20):2674–9.

23. Qi H, Li S. Dose-response meta-analysis on coffee, tea and caffeine consumption with risk of Parkinson's disease. Geriatr Gerontol Int 2014;14(2):430–9.
24. Ascherio A, Chen H, Schwarzschild MA, et al. Caffeine, postmenopausal estrogen, and risk of Parkinson's disease. Neurology 2003;60(5):790–5.
25. Postuma RB, Lang AE, Munhoz RP, et al. Caffeine for treatment of Parkinson disease: a randomized controlled trial. Neurology 2012;79(7):651–8.
26. Wills AM, Eberly S, Tennis M, et al. Caffeine consumption and risk of dyskinesia in CALM-PD. Mov Disord 2013;28:380–3.
27. Postuma RB, Anang J, Pelletier A, et al. Caffeine as symptomatic treatment for Parkinson disease (Café-PD): a randomized trial. Neurology 2017;89(17): 1795–803.
28. Jaussent I, Dauvilliers Y, Ancelin ML, et al. Insomnia symptoms in older adults: associated factors and gender differences. Am J Geriatr Psychiatry 2011;19(1): 88–97.
29. Clark I, Landolt HP. Coffee, caffeine, and sleep: a systematic review of epidemiological studies and randomized controlled trials. Sleep Med Rev 2017;31:70–8.
30. Patel D, Steinberg J, Patel P. Insomnia in the elderly: a review. J Clin Sleep Med 2018;14(6):1017–24.
31. Jaussent I, Bouyer J, Ancelin ML, et al. Insomnia and daytime sleepiness are risk factors for depressive symptoms in the elderly. Sleep 2011;34(8):1103–10.
32. Frozi J, de Carvalho HW, Ottoni GL, et al. Distinct sensitivity to caffeine-induced insomnia related to age. J Psychopharmacol 2018;32(1):89–95.
33. Farazdaq H, Andrades M, Nanji K. Insomnia and its correlates among elderly patients presenting to family medicine clinics at an academic center. Malays Fam Physician 2018;13(3):12–9.
34. Hu Y, Stephenson K, Klare D. The dynamic relationship between daily caffeine intake and sleep duration in middle-aged and older adults. J Sleep Res 2020; 29(6):e12996.
35. Martyn D, Lau A, Richardson P, et al. Temporal patterns of caffeine intake in the United States. Food Chem Toxicol 2018;111:71–83.
36. Okun M, Reynolds CF, Buysse DJ, et al. Sleep variability, health-related practices and inflammatory markers in a community dwelling sample of older adults. Psychosom Med 2011;73(2):142–50.
37. Furman D, Chang J, Lartigue L, et al. Expression of specific inflammasome gene modules stratifies older individuals into two extreme clinical and immunological states. Nat Med 2017;23(2):174–84.
38. Robillard R, Bouchard M, Cartier A, et al. Sleep is more sensitive to high doses of caffeine in the middle years of life. J Psychopharmacol 2015;29(6):688–97.
39. Aziz R, Steffens DC. What are the causes of late-life depression? Psychiatr Clin North Am 2013;36(4):497–516.
40. Wang L, Shen X, Wu Y, et al. Coffee and caffeine consumption and depression: a meta-analysis of observational studies. Aust N Z J Psychiatry 2016;50(3):228–42.
41. Aggarwal R, Kunik M, Asghar-Ali A. Anxiety in later life. Focus (Am Psychiatr Publ) 2017;15(2):157–61.
42. Pary R, Sarai SK, Micchelli A, et al. Anxiety disorders in older patients. Prim Care Companion CNS Disord 2019;21(1):18nr02335.
43. Dada F, Sethi S, Grossberg GT. Generalized anxiety disorder in the elderly. Psychiatr Clin North Am 2001;24(1):155–64.
44. Pan CW, Ma Q, Sun HP, et al. Tea consumption and health-related quality of life in older adults. J Nutr Health Aging 2017;21(5):480–6.

45. Feng L, Yan Z, Sun B, et al. Tea consumption and depressive symptoms in older people in rural China. J Am Geriatr Soc 2013;61(11):1943–7.
46. Kim J, Kim J. Green tea, coffee, and caffeine consumption are inversely associated with self-report lifetime depression in the Korean population. Nutrients 2018; 10(9):1201.
47. Kimura Y, Suga H, Kobayashi S, et al. Three-Generation Study of Women on Diets and Health Study Group. Intake of coffee associated with decreased depressive symptoms among elderly Japanese women: a multi-center cross-sectional study. J Epidemiol 2020;30(8):338–44.
48. Iranpour S, Sabour S. Inverse association between caffeine intake and depressive symptoms in US adults: data from National Health and Nutrition Examination Survey (NHANES) 2005-2006. Psychiatry Res 2019;271:732–9.
49. Lucas M, Mirzaei F, Pan A, et al. Coffee, caffeine, and risk of depression among women. Arch Intern Med 2011;171(17):1571–8.
50. Guo X, Park Y, Freedman ND, et al. Sweetened beverages, coffee, and tea and depression risk among older US adults. PLoS One 2014;9(4):e94715.
51. Hall S, Desbrow B, Anoopkumar-Dukie S, et al. A review of the bioactivity of coffee, caffeine and key coffee constituents on inflammatory responses linked to depression. Food Res Int 2015;76(3):626–36.
52. Rycerz K, Jaworska-Adamu JE. Effects of aspartame metabolites on astrocytes and neurons. Folia Neuropathol 2013;51(1):10–7.
53. Polasek TM, Patel F, Jensen BP, et al. Predicted metabolic drug clearance with increasing adult age. Br J Clin Pharmacol 2013;75(4):1019–28.
54. Nehlig A. Interindividual differences in caffeine metabolism and factors driving caffeine consumption. Pharmacol Rev 2018;70(2):384–411.
55. Carrillo JA, Benitez J. Clinically significant pharmacokinetic interactions between dietary caffeine and medications. Clin Pharmacokinet 2000;39(2):127–53.
56. Broderick PJ, Benjamin AB, Dennis LW. Caffeine and psychiatric medication interactions: a review. J Okla State Med Assoc 2005;98(8):380–4.
57. Myslobodsky M. The paradox of caffeine-zolpidem interaction: a network analysis. Curr Drug Targets 2009;10(10):1009–20.

Applying Geriatric Principles to Hazardous Drinking in Older Adults

Miriam B. Rodin, MD, PhD

KEYWORDS

- Older adults • Polypharmacy • Frailty • Unsafe drinking • Hazardous drinking
- Alcohol use disorder • Annual medicare wellness • Alcohol intervention

KEY POINTS

- The concept of hazardous drinking addresses the risks of alcohol consumption in older adults that may not fit the DSM-5 AUD criteria.
- The interplay of ethanol with physiological changes of aging, comorbidity and polypharmacy increases risk for falls, traffic accidents, drug interactions and victimization.
- Increased numbers of older adults and increased proportions of older adults who continue to drink warrants clinical vigilance.
- Routine office visits and the Medicare Annual Wellness Visit are opportunities to screen using short, validated tools such as the AUDIT-C and the SASQ.
- Always consider alcohol or benzodiazepine withdrawal in hospitalized older adults who become delirious.

INTRODUCTION

For many older adults, alcohol is an adjunct to family celebrations and other social engagement that is important to their sense of well-being.[1,2] Recently a respected Washington political columnist wrote his reflections on reaching the age of 80 years and complained about his doctors lecturing him about his evening martini.[3] We need to understand in our patients and our society that having a drink is not inherently good or bad or unhealthy. There are guidelines for safe drinking and red flags that any clinician caring for older adults should recognize. This article will focus on recognizing and distinguishing potentially unhealthy alcohol intake in older adults from alcohol use disorder (AUD) and summarize approaches to counseling older adults for safe drinking and treatment of AUD.

Division of Geriatric Medicine, Department of Internal Medicine, St. Louis University School of Medicine, SLUCare Academic Pavilion, 1008 South Spring Avenue 2nd Floor, St Louis, MO 63110, USA
E-mail address: miriam.rodin@health.slu.edu
Twitter: @Rodin4M (M.B.R.)

Clin Geriatr Med 38 (2022) 145–158
https://doi.org/10.1016/j.cger.2021.08.001
0749-0690/22/© 2021 Elsevier Inc. All rights reserved.

EPIDEMIOLOGY OF DRINKING AND POLYPHARMACY

Alcohol has been around for a long time. Over the past century, the age at first alcohol use has trended to younger ages, now averaging about 25 years.[4–8] Among those older than 65 years, drinking declines with age. Among those older than 85 years, fewer than 5% continue to drink. Surveys find risky drinking in the single digits among adults older than 75 years. Clinical samples in outpatient clinics[9–11] and emergency departments[12,13] have a selection bias for higher drinking, but even there, the proportion of older adults in the trauma bay is small.[14–16] Older adults are also using both recreational and prescription substances.[4,17–19] The general caution should be that all health surveys of older adults suffer from survivor bias.[20,21] Older adults who continue to drink say that they drink less not for health reasons but rather for lack of opportunity, lack of access, and direct concern about drug interactions.[1,16,22,23]

Polypharmacy is problematic for older adults with multiple comorbidities. Between 26% to 40% of Medicare age adults are at risk of adverse drug interactions simply because of numbers of prescription and over the counter (OTC) drugs they take.[24–27] Older adults are more likely to get new prescriptions for opiates[25,26,28,29] and benzodiazepines.[30] Other risky drugs more frequently prescribed to older adults include muscle relaxants, antidepressants, antihistamines, anticholinergics, antihypertensives, and hypoglycemic drugs.[24]

THE PHARMACOLOGY, CHEMISTRY, AND PHYSIOLOGY OF ETHANOL

Ethanol is absorbed directly from the upper gastrointestinal (GI) tract, metabolized in the liver by alcohol dehydrogenase (ADH) and, to some extent, by the cytochrome P450 CYP-2E1 that also metabolizes fatty acids. The first 2 steps reduce ethanol back to acetaldehyde and ultimately to CO_2 and H_2O. There are many genetically determined variants of both enzymes, so there is great individual variability in the rate of metabolism and subjective response to and excretion of ethanol.[31]

Ethanol is a naturally occurring chemical that is used as a drug. Pharmacokinetic studies have examined how ethanol interacts with drugs using a variety of designs. A systematic review concluded that due to factors of variable study design, small numbers and unmeasured subject genetic variability, prior ethanol exposures, and multidrug interactions, it is difficult to identify specific drug-ethanol interaction effects based on kinetics. The literature is more consistent about the pharmacodynamic, or subjective, effects of ethanol with other drugs. There were consistent additive effects on symptoms such as subjective intoxication, sedation, hypertension, psychomotor performance impairment, blood pressure, and heart rate when ethanol was given with a target drug.[32] With aging, the volume of distribution decreases, so equivalent servings of alcohol produce higher blood levels faster in older drinkers. Age- or disease-related decreased liver enzyme (ADH, CYP-450-2E1) activity and decreased renal clearance increase alcohol blood levels and delay its clearance in women and older drinkers. Interplay with genetic variability, sex, age-related changes in central nervous system (CNS) function, and additive effects of other drugs make for a complicated picture. **Table 1** shows, for example, the ten drugs most often prescribed to older adults in the United States (U.S.) with potential alcohol interactions.

Ethanol has both acute and chronic toxicity. The metabolite acetaldehyde independently causes subjectively unpleasant flushing and sweating in some drinkers. Alcohol can induce direct irritation and inflammation in the upper GI tract. It binds avidly to the inhibitory neurotransmitter gamma-butyric acid receptors in the CNS, but it also indirectly stimulates the mu and dopamine receptor reward systems. This poses a

Table 1
Interaction of ethanol with the ten most frequently prescribed drugs in the elderly

Drug	Indication	Metabolism	Potential Ethanol Interaction
Simvastatin	Hyperlipidemia, atherosclerosis, diabetes (DM)	Liver CYP 450:2D6, 3A4 Inhibits cholesterol synthesis	Caution in alcohol use due to liver enzyme elevations
Lisinopril	Hypertension (HTN), congestive heart failure (CHF)	None, inhibits ACE conversion of angiotensin 1 to angiotensin 2.	Hypotension
Levothyroxine	Hypothyroidism	Metabolized in liver unknown pathway	None known
Amlodipine besylate	Hypertension (HTN)	Liver CYP450: 3A4	Hypotension
Omeprazole	Acid reflux	Liver CYP 450: 2C19, 3A4	None known
Azithromycin	Antibiotic, pneumonia, bronchitis	Liver	None known
Metformin	Type 2 diabetes	None	Inhibits hepatic gluconeogenesis, prolongs hypoglycemia, increases risk for lactic acidosis.
Amoxacillin	Antibiotic	Limited, excreted in urine	None direct
Hydrochlorothiazide	Diuretic, HTN, CHF	None	Hypotension
Hydrocodone	Pain	Liver extensive CYP450: 2D6, 3A4	Coingestion raises hydrocodone levels additive risk of respiratory depression, sedation, psychomotor impairment, hypotension. In combination with acetaminophen increased liver toxicity

particular risk for older drinkers who experience disturbances of attention and coordination at blood levels much lower than required to impair younger drinkers.[16,33,34]

Alcohol is a depressant, so after a first pleasant euphoria at high blood levels, it causes sedation, coma, and death. Ethanol antagonizes the excitatory transmitter glutamate from binding with N-Methyl-D-Aspartate (NMDA) receptors. Under the influence of continuous suppression by daily drinking, glutamate receptors multiply creating the substrate for withdrawal syndromes including catecholamine rebound tachycardia, hypertension, hallucinosis, seizures, and delirium.[33] Mortality from delirium tremens, the most severe withdrawal syndrome, has declined with improved recognition and management, but it remains deadly for older adults.[12]

ASSESSING DRINKING SAFETY FOR OLDER ADULTS

The terms "problem drinking", "alcohol abuse", and "alcohol dependence" have been replaced in the diagnostic and statistical manual (DSM)-5 with "substance use disorder" which includes 10 classes of ingestible or injectable substances.[35] The DSM-5 defines substance use disorders as continuing to use a substance after experiencing problems either caused by or associated with use. This is distinguished from substance-induced disorders such as hallucinations or withdrawal syndromes. Eleven criteria in 4 domains of adverse substance use apply to drinking as well and are linked to altered activation of the brain's intrinsic reward system. **Boxes 1** and **2** show the 11 criteria and scoring system used to diagnose AUD. The DSM-5 also recognizes substance-induced psychiatric disorders including depression, anxiety, psychosis, obsessional-compulsive disorders, neurocognitive disorders, sleep disorders, sexual disfunction, and delirium. These disorders are distinct from intoxications and withdrawal syndromes.

A newer concept is "at-risk" or "unhealthy"[36] or "hazardous" alcohol use which is defined as consumption of any amount of alcohol that may result in adverse effects and does not fit criteria for a diagnosis of AUD. Based on epidemiologic studies, multiple public health authorities including the National Institute on Alcohol Abuse and Alcoholism, Centers for Disease Control and Prevention, Surgeon General, and US Preventive Services Task Force (USPSTF) (2018)[37] have agreed on safe levels of alcohol intake for

---

Box 1
DSM-5 criteria for alcohol use disorder

1. Uncontrolled use
   1. Drinking more or for longer than intended
   2. Repeated unsuccessful attempts to cut back or control drinking

2. Continued use despite consequences
   3. Social problems (job problems) caused or exacerbated by use
   4. Using alcohol in physically hazardous settings
   5. Medical or psychological problems caused or worsened by drinking

3. More time spent on alcohol
   6. A great deal of time spent using, obtaining or recovering from alcohol
   7. Have given up important things or cut back on previously important, enjoyable things because of drinking
   8. Failure to fulfill major obligations (work, family, relationships) due to drinking

4. Biological responses
   9. Craving, thinking about it a lot, missing the sensations
   10. Tolerance, takes more to get the same level of positive sensation
   11. Withdrawal symptoms, shakiness, seizures, nausea, vomiting, tachycardia, and hallucinations on stopping

Scoring:
  Mild AUD 2 to 4
  Moderate AUD4-5
  Severe AUD $\geq$ 6

Data from DSM-5 Task Force C, Diagnostic and Statistical Manual of the American Psychiatric Association. Fifth ed. 2013. Arlington, VA.

Box 2

Unhealthy drinking National Institute on Alcohol Abuse and Alcoholism guidelines for adults: drinks per week, per day

Daily limits for men ≤5, for older men greater than 4

Daily limits for women ≤4, for older women ≤3

Weekly limits for men ≤14 Weekly limits for women ≤7

Alcohol equivalents: 1 drink = one 12-oz bottle or glass of beer, one 5-oz glass of wine, one 1.5-oz shot of liquor

---

the general adult population and issued a modified recommendation for older adults. **Boxes 1 and 2** additionally show the current guidelines for safe drinking in adults.

The risk in "at-risk" drinking includes the drinker and a spouse who is also at risk due to disability, frailty, and cognitive impairment. Alcohol is implicated in geriatric trauma including traffic, occupational, firearm, and household accidents. Older drinkers in motor vehicle accidents have lower blood alcohol concentration than younger drivers involved in traffic fatalities. Polypharmacy exacerbates the risk of hemodynamic, glycemic, and cognitive events. The interaction of small amounts of cannabis and alcohol is of increasing concern as both are legal and widely available without prescription. The ability to compensate for alcohol is affected by how many small deficits an older adult has accumulated, a well-accepted principle in geriatric medicine.[38] The idea of aging itself as the accumulation of decreased organ reserve and decreased ability to restore homeostasis is especially pertinent for older people who drink.[39] The subclinical markers of frailty that can be detected by a thorough geriatric examination can identify "vulnerabilities" to the effects of ethanol on older adults.

HOW TO RECOGNIZE UNSAFE DRINKING IN OLDER ADULTS

Unsafe drinking and AUD are different conditions in older adults. Cutoffs derived from a population survey found that greater than 1 drink per day, greater than 7 drinks per week, or ≥3 drinks on any occasion predicted alcohol-related problems in middle-aged drinkers. At 10-year follow-up, when they were 65 to 75 years old, most of the daily drinkers had cut down or stopped. But even at the same levels of drinking, older drinkers experienced fewer of the 11 alcohol-related problems detailed in the DSM-5 criteria than the younger drinkers.[40] Although fewer than 20% of those over 70 drink, the consequences are serious enough to warrant screening older adults who can answer for themselves. Several screening tools identify AUD. The Alcohol Use Disorders Identification Test (AUDIT) is a 10-item questionnaire widely used in English and translations.[41] The AUDIT-C short form is used as a first-level screen. It is limited to the first 3 quantity/frequency items which were adopted in setting the safe levels referenced previously. The Single Alcohol Screening Questionnaire (SASQ) about having 5 or more drinks on one occasion in the past year has been shown to identify hazardous drinking in outpatient settings. The 4-item Cut-down, Annoyed, Guilty, Eye-opener (CAGE) and the 24-item Michigan Alcohol Screening Test (MAST-G)[42] also screen for AUD. The AUDIT-C is a less intimidating way to open the conversation at least for initial interviews in a primary care setting. The MAST-G recognizes that older adults are likely to be retired, so there are fewer employment-related consequences. They are more likely to be unpartnered, so there are fewer people be annoyed by their drinking.[36,43]

CLINICAL APPROACHES TO ALCOHOL IN OLDER ADULTS IN OUTPATIENT CARE

Alcohol, tobacco, and off-prescription addictive or recreational drug use are subsumed under social history in many electronic medical records. This is unfortunate because it encourages a superficial approach to important health-related behaviors, exposures, and social risk. The Annual Medicare Wellness (AMW) visit provides clinicians with an opportunity to screen for harmful alcohol use. Pathways for screening and intervention in primary care have described and evaluated.[43] Alcohol abstinence on a screening tool may be a marker of previous problems with alcohol. Nondrinkers should be asked how long they have been abstinent or if they just never drank. Adult-onset abstinence should prompt a query about reasons for stopping. Previous heavy drinking may have contributed to their current comorbidities involving heart, liver, pancreas, trauma, and neurologic function. Current or previous heavy alcohol use may identify comorbid psychiatric illnesses and family dysfunction. The Review of Symptoms offers another opportunity to identify alcohol effects especially urinary frequency and sleep complaints. Screening for depression is part of an AMW.[29,43] Higher than recommended alcohol intake even in the absence of a formal AUD diagnosis can be associated with other off-prescription substance use. Older adults should be asked about other drugs. The decision to prescribe narcotics or benzodiazepines should be carefully evaluated in patients with at-risk alcohol use.

The drug review at every geriatric clinic visit is one of the most important medical procedures to be offered. It reveals adherence or nonadherence, identifies other prescribers, and facilitates drug reconciliation and deprescribing based on the STOPP-START principle.[44] Medication review should always include OTC medications and nutraceuticals. Medication review and reconciliation provides a platform to discuss actual or potential drug-alcohol interactions and provides a clear rationale for counseling.[28]

Patients who trigger concern for hazardous drinking or AUD should be evaluated using more in-depth questionnaires such as the full AUDIT, CAGE, or others. Hazardous drinking may not need a formal outpatient or inpatient rehabilitation approach. If the clinician is comfortable with an office-based intervention, several authorities recommended proceeding to the Brief Negotiated Interview (BNI).[45] The BNI starts with the clinician stating their concern and requesting the patient's permission to discuss their drinking. The clinician inquires about the patient's perception of their drinking. If there is agreement about the concern, the patient can be engaged to identify a change they would be willing to make to enhance their health. The BNI has 7 steps:

1. Establish rapport with the patient.
2. Explore their views about pros and cons of changing their alcohol drinking.
3. Review the health risks of continued drinking.
4. Summarize and ask whether they think a change is needed.
5. Explore readiness, that is, what things they would need to do to change their drinking.
6. Identify a goal.
7. Explore their confidence that they can do it.

The BNI constitutes the first step of the Screening Brief Intervention Referral to Treatment (SBIRT) structured approach to alcohol intervention.[46]

CASE 1: A 70-YEAR-OLD MARRIED MAN

The patient was seen virtually for his AMW visit. There have been no changes in his state of health. His review of systems (ROS) is negative.

His medications are amlodipine, losartan, hydrochlorothiazide, tamsulosin, atorvastatin, and aspirin. His rapid geriatric assessment (RGA) indicates no concerns regarding nutrition, gait and balance, depression, or cognition.[47]

Social History

He enjoys going on cruises with his wife and is looking forward to "when all this (Covid) is over." He does not smoke or use other substances. On AUDIT-C, he reports he has always had a couple drinks before dinner, occasionally more if out with friends. He denies ever having more than 5 drinks on any occasion in the past year. When he has been drinking, he states his wife is the "designated driver." But with Covid, that has not happened lately. In follow-up, SASQ was rephrased as "ever." He says he has had episodes of greater than recommended drinking before Covid.

Assessment

He does not trigger either AUD or hazardous intake for age. But it is borderline and possibly situational.

Intervention

We engaged in a brief motivational interview about drinking safely "when things open up again." He agrees to revisit the subject at his next annual examination. He is advised to increase his exercise.

This case illustrates a man whose drinking is within recommended levels, but there is a small concern regarding his past intake and the effects of increased opportunities for socializing. If AUD or hazardous drinking is identified during his follow-up visit, the previous SBIRT can be recalled and reviewed. This patient does not appear to need referral to a specialized treatment program.[48]

TREATMENT MODALITIES

The success of multimodal interventions depends in part on how the patient identifies goals of abstinence, low risk drinking or no goal.[49] Multimodal programs have shown equivalent efficacy in older adults.[49] Abstinence is not necessarily the goal of all treatment programs, but patients who set the goal of abstinence tend to do better. Interventions with patients suffering from AUD should be multimodal. The evidence for outpatient cognitive behavioral therapy (CBT) alone is not convincing.[50] Examples of psychosocial interventions include CBT, motivational interviewing to promote change, and mutual help groups including but not limited to Alcoholics Anonymous. Participating in more than one treatment modality appears to promote patients' adherence to their goals. The COMBINE trial compared medical management with naltrexone or acamprosate or both or neither with Combination Behavioral Intervention (CBI) with medical management or alone, a six-arm trial. Only the naltrexone combined with CBI achieved significant resolution of heavy drinking. A caveat is that median age of the 1383 subjects was 44 years.[51] There are few studies of AUD treatment either focusing on or including enough older drinkers to make an aging-specific recommendation. But a meta-analysis is encouraging.[49]

Medication-assisted treatment for all substance use disorders has been increasing. This includes AUD. There are 5 available drugs shown in **Table 2**: naltrexone, acamprosate, disulfiram, topiramate, and gabapentin. There are few head-to-head trials, but all have shown efficacy in decreasing heavy drinking. Evidence for baclofen is uncertain.[52] When caring for an older adult with AUD, the choice of the drug depends on potential interactions with other drugs they are taking, renal and liver function, ability to manage their own medications, and cost. Disulfiram is contraindicated in older adults because of the severity of adverse reactions if they do drink or accidently use mouth wash or cough syrup with alcohol. Naltrexone is effective and relatively free of adverse

Table 2
Pharmacotherapy options for treating AUB in older adults

Indication	FDA Approved	FDA Approved	FDA Approved	Off Label	Off Label
Drug	Disulfiram	Acamprosate	Naltrexone	Topiramate	Gabapentin
Mechanism of action	Inhibits enzyme acetaldehyde dehydrogenase	Unknown, affects interaction between gamma-butyric acid (GABA) and glutamate	Opiate antagonist	GABA agonist, glutamate antagonist, inhibits carbonic anhydrase, antiepileptic activity.	Modulates glutamate release, antiepileptic activity
Safety concerns	Alcohol ingestion triggers flushing, tachycardia, nausea, vomiting. May be severe. May be triggered by other drugs, for example, metronidazole	Should not be used in depression, suicidality, renal CrCl<30	Should not be used if taking opioids for pain or in substance abuse management without consultation.	Should not be used if actively drinking, taking metformin, glaucoma depression or suicidality.	Should not be used if taking opioids, caution with liver, renal impairment Can be sedating.
Comorbidity/ polypharmacy concerns	Heart disease	Renal failure, depression screening, other antiepileptic, neuropathy medications	None specific after opiate screening, medication review	Diabetes, history psychiatric illness, glaucoma, verify psychiatric, diabetic, and glaucoma medications	Commonly used in treatment of neuropathy, verify current medications
Community pharmacy cost (GoodRx)	$40/mo	$80/mo	PO $30/mo IM $1200/mo including adm	$20	$10/mo

drug interactions in older adults. However, as many older adults have been prescribed narcotic analgesics, this should be done only after narcotics have been withdrawn. If pain cannot be managed without narcotics, one of the other drugs could be considered.[49,52]

Referral to outpatient multimodal therapy may tax an older person's transportation system, especially if driving is a concern. An additional consideration in caring for an older adult with AUD are comorbid medical conditions, visual and hearing impairment, mobility, cognitive status, comorbid psychiatric diagnoses, and cognitive impairment. The family of older drinkers may include adult children who need to be mobilized in support of the older drinker or counseled for their own trauma as survivors of family dysfunction related to the drinker.

CASE 2: AN 83-YEAR-OLD WIDOWED MAN

The patient came alone to a *routine follow up in the clinic*. He has no new complaints. On *ROS*, he continues to complain about difficulty falling asleep. He is bothered by urinary frequency. He denies short of breath, chest pain, weight loss, or falls. He recently experienced sudden loss of vision in one eye.

His medications reflect his significant cardiac history: lisinopril, carvedilol, simvastatin, clopidogrel, aspirin, levothyroxine, tamsulosin, mirabegron, diazepam 5 mg at night for sleep, apixaban, metformin, glargine, and omeprazole. His office HbA1c was 10.9 indicating poor adherence to diabetes management.

His *social history* is remarkable for having a highly successful business career. His wife passed away several years ago, and he misses her very much. He used to play golf, but his vision and low back pain do not permit it anymore. He never smoked. AUDIT-C revealed he has "a couple of drinks" in the evening to help him sleep. He goes to his private club once a week but stated he never has more than 2 drinks with his friends. When asked how far away his club is from his home, he states it is "a couple of miles" so he drives. He generally goes in the evening to avoid rush hour.

On *physical examination*, he is alert and able to state date, place and situation. RGA revealed mild dementia (SLUMS 25/30). His gait is broad-based but steady. He does not use a cane. He screened negative for depression and nutritional risk. He has movement-only vision in his left eye and wears a hearing aid on the right.

Assessment

Assessments involded polypharmacy including several drugs with potential ethanol interaction, anticoagulants, metformin, insulin, antihypertensives, and a nonanticholinergic medication for urinary incontinence. His use of a long-acting benzodiazepine is worrisome. He denies any heavy drinking. He denies falls.

Intervention

When counseled to cut down or stop drinking, he is not agreeable to further discussion about his drinking, but he does agree to stop driving because of his poor vision. He gives the clinician permission to call his son to report concerns.

At a *second appointment*, the father and son were asked to come together. His son reports significantly heavier drinking than the patient admits and multiple falls. A diagnosis of AUD is made. Although the depression screening responses are negative, his son reports that his father has been quite alone since his wife died and he talks about missing her often. The patient was not agreeable to a psychiatry referral. The patient did agree to prescription of an antidepressant, mirtazapine, and tapering the benzodiazepine. However, his medication adherence was not certain. His son agreed to visit daily to give him his medications until he could arrange with a home care agency to provide a companion and medication supervision. The father and son agreed to discuss a senior living community nearer to the son where he will have more socialization. The patient and his son agreed to return in a month to review their progress and reconsider a referral to outpatient psychiatry to treat depression.

Another consideration in older adults as well as any older substance users is the network of support they have. For older adults, as seen in case #2, the patient has a son who is willing to support his AUD treatment. Owing to vision and hearing loss, it is doubtful the patient could manage multimodal outpatient therapy. With better supervision, risk for falls, diabetic control, and transportation can be addressed. Caregivers vary in their ability to recognize the problem and their own resources to intervene. The prevalence of psychiatric comorbidity in actively drinking older adults can lead to additional safety concerns besides falls, motor vehicle accidents, and suicide.

CASE 3: A DIVORCED 69-YEAR-OLD WOMAN

The patient had previously lived with her daughter in another city. When that daughter died, her other daughter brought the patient to live with her. She was *seen in the clinic several weeks later to establish care and to obtain a referral to psychiatry*. The daughter knew very little about the medical history, but she had been treated for schizophrenia much of her life. The daughter did not know what medications she took and had none with her at the visit. On *social history*, the daughter reported smoking tobacco and cannabis and was very concerned about her drinking. The clinician asked how the patient got the drugs and alcohol. The daughter reported that the patient walked to the corner store while she was at work and bought a six-pack of beer mostly every day and some marijuana if one the men was selling. She typically drank "a six-pack" a day.

On *physical examination*, the patient was not cooperative. She was agitated and difficult to redirect. She stated clearly that she did not want to be there. She did not have severe cognitive impairment. She could rapidly say the months of the year backward; she was oriented to person, place, day, date, time, and situation. She appeared to be at least her stated age. She got up several times to leave, using a wheeled walker to go out in the hall. She was reluctant to try to walk without it.

Assessment

The first concern is to establish psychiatric care and provide supervision. Her drinking is hazardous because it exceeds safe amounts. Her fall risk is increased by gait instability and cannabis use. She is a target for street crime when she goes out alone using a walker to buy beer and pot. The daughter is unable to provide supervision because she needs to work. During Covid, senior day cares were closed, but it is likely that day care would depend on better management of her psychiatric symptoms.

Intervention

The daughter refused direct hospital admission for psychiatric stabilization. The most urgent issue besides psychiatric stabilization is the lack of supervision. The daughter was informed that her mother was unable to care for herself in her present condition. She is in danger when she goes out alone with cash to buy pot and alcohol on the corner. This could be reported as neglect to the state department on aging. A social work organization was consulted to initiate home services. The daughter was assisted by social work to complete the Family Medical Leave Act forms to be excused from work by her employer while attending the patient's urgent medical needs. She agreed to have a caregiver while she was at work and to leave no cash, cards, or alcohol in the home. Psychiatry referral was placed to establish psychiatric care as soon as possible. If the patient was in fact drinking a six-pack of beer a day, withdrawal seemed possible. The daughter was instructed to recognize those signs and call emergency medical services. Shortly thereafter, the patient was admitted through the emergency department at another hospital. From there, she was discharged to a long-term care facility.

SUMMARY AND CONCLUSIONS

Geriatricians and other primary care clinicians should follow the USPSTF guidelines for safe drinking for older adults. If screening with a short form such as the AUDIT-C suggests a potential for risky drinking, it is recommended to start a conversation with the patient. If RGA indicates frailty, depression, malnutrition, increased fall risk, or cognitive impairment, a caregiver or family member should be engaged, with permission, in the discussion of hazardous drinking. Polypharmacy should prompt a review using the STOPP-START principles. The RGA may uncover additional obstacles to multimodal interventions. Multimodal interventions for frail older drinkers should also include geriatric interventions including mobilization of caregivers, support for caregivers, home health services, medication supervision, and falls prevention. The SBIRT cycle has been successful with cognitively intact older adults although there are few dedicated studies. Multimodal interventions are generally more effective than individual counseling. Pharmacotherapy should not be overlooked for selected older drinkers. However, adding another drug to polypharmacy requires a cautious approach. Clinicians who are not confident or experienced in managing AUD (or polysubstance abuse of any form) should promptly refer to specialty care.

CLINICS CARE POINTS

- Older adults should be asked if they consume alcohol and if yes, use one of the short validated screening tools to assess potential risk. eg, excessive quantity, driving, falls.
- Review the medication list for potentially hazardous pharmacologic interactions and advise or deprescribe accordingly.
- Brief interventions including motivational interviewing may be effective for reducing hazardous drinking.
- If drinking patterns suggest an alcohol use disorder referral to treatment is advisable.

DISCLOSURE

The author has nothing to disclose.

REFERENCES

1. Scott R, Wiener CH, Paulson D, et al. Functional limitation in later-life: the impact of sips, socialization and sadness. Aging Ment Health 2020;2:107.
2. van Gils Y, Dom G, Dierckx E, et al. Resilience, depression and anxiety and hazardous alcohol use behaviour among community dwelling older adults. Aging Ment Health 2021;1–9.
3. Will, George. What my 80 years have taught me. Opinion. Washington Post Available at: https://www.washngtonpost.com/opinions. Accessed May 7, 2021.

4. Wang YP, Andrade LH. Epidemiology of alcohol and drug use in the elderly. Curr Opin Psychiatry 2013;26(4):343–8.

5. Frisher M, Mendonça M, Shelton N, et al. Is alcohol consumption in older adults associated with poor self-rated health? Cross-sectional and longitudinal analyses from the English Longitudinal Study of Ageing. BMC Public Health 2015;15:703.

6. Ahlner F, Sigström R, Rydberg Sterner T, et al. Increased alcohol consumption among Swedish 70-year-olds 1976 to 2016: analysis of data from the gothenburg H70 birth cohort studies, Sweden. Alcohol Clin Exp Res 2018;42(12):2403–12.

7. Tyrovolas S, Panaretos D, Daskalopoulou C, et al. Alcohol drinking and health in ageing: a global scale analysis of older individual data through the harmonised dataset of ATHLOS. Nutrients 2020;12(6):1746.

8. van den Brandt PA, Brandts L. Alcohol consumption in later life and reaching longevity: The Netherlands Cohort Study. Age Ageing 2020;49(3):395–402.

9. Sterling A, Palzes VA, Lu Y, et al. Associations between medical conditions and alcohol consumption levels in an adult primary care population. JAMA Netw Open 2020;3(5):e204687.

10. Zanjani F, Smith R, Slavova S, et al. Concurrent alcohol and medication poisoning hospital admissions among older rural and urban residents. Am J Drug Alcohol Abuse 2016;42(4):422–30.

11. Joseph CL, Ganzini L, Atkinson RM. Screening for alcohol use disorders in the nursing home. J Am Geriatr Soc 1995;43(4):368–73.

12. Salottolo K, McGuire E, Mains CW, et al. Occurrence, predictors, and prognosis of alcohol withdrawal syndrome and delirium tremens following traumatic injury. Crit Care Med 2017;45(5):867–74.

13. Qian XX, Chau PH, Kwan CW, et al. Investigating risk factors for falls among community-dwelling older adults according to WHO's risk factor model for falls. J Nutr Health Aging 2021;25(4):425–32.

14. Scheetz LJ. One for the road: a comparison of drinking and driving behavior among younger and older adults involved in fatal crashes. J Trauma Nurs 2015;22(4):187–93.

15. Chippendale T, Gentile PA, James MK. Characteristics and consequences of falls among older adult trauma patients: considerations for injury prevention programs. Aust Occup Ther J 2017;64(5):350–7.

16. Price JL, Lewis B, Boissoneualt J, et al. Effects of acute alcohol and driving complexity in older and younger adults. Psychopharmacology (Berl.) 2018; 235(3):887–96.

17. Wu LT, Blazer DG. Illicit and nonmedical drug use among older adults: a review. J Aging Health 2011;23(3):481–504.

18. Fairman KA, Early NK. Treatment needs and service utilization in older U.S. Adults evidencing high-risk substance use. J Aging Health 2020;32(10):1363–75.

19. Barry KL, Blow FC. Drinking over the Lifespan: focus on older adults. Alcohol Res 2016;38(1):115–20.

20. Kelfve S, Ahacic K. Bias in estimates of alcohol use among older people: selection effects due to design, health, and cohort replacement. BMC Public Health 2015;15:769.

21. Tolvanen E, Seppa K, Lintonen T, et al. Old people, alcohol use and mortality. A ten-prospective study. Aging Clin Exp Res 2005;17(5):426–33.

22. Matthews DB, Schneider A, Kastner A, et al. I can't drink what I used to: the interaction between ethanol and the aging brain. Int Rev Neurobiol 2019;148:79–99.

23. Soler-Vila H, Ortolá R, García-Esquinas E, et al. Changes in alcohol consumption and associated variables among older adults in Spain: a population-based cohort study. Sci Rep 2019;9(1):10401.

24. Immonen S, Valvanne J, Pitkälä KH, et al. The prevalence of potential alcohol-drug interactions in older adults. Scand J Prim Health Care 2013;31(2):73–8.

25. Cousins G, Galvin R, Flood M, et al. Potential for alcohol and drug interactions in older adults: evidence from the Irish longitudinal study on ageing. BMC Geriatr 2014;14:57.

26. Holton AE, Gallagher P, Fahey T, et al. Concurrent use of alcohol interactive medications and alcohol in older adults: a systematic review of prevalence and associated adverse outcomes. BMC Geriatr 2017;17(1):148.

27. Holton A, Boland F, Gallagher P, et al. Longitudinal prevalence of potentially serious alcohol-medication interactions in community-dwelling older adults: a prospective cohort study. Eur J Clin Pharmacol 2019;75(4):569–75.

28. Qato DM, Manzoor BS, Lee TA, et al. Drug-alcohol interactions in older U.S. Adults. J Am Geriatr Soc 2015;63(11):2324–31.

29. Britton A, Fat LN, Neligan A, et al. The association between alcohol consumption and sleep disorders among older people in the general population. Sci Rep 2020; 10(1):5275.

30. Maust DT, Kales HC, Wiechers IR, et al. No end in sight: benzodiazepine use in older adults in the United States. J Am Geriatr Soc 2016;64(12):2546–53.

31. Cederbaum AI. Alcohol metabolism. Clin Liver Dis 2012;16(4):667–85.

32. Chan L-N, Anderson GD. Pharmacokinetic and pharmacodynamic drug interactions with ethanol (alcohol). Clin Pharmacokinet 2014;53(12):1115–36.

33. Lewis B, Garcia CC, Boissoneault J, et al. Working memory performance following acute alcohol: replication and extension of dose by age interactions. J Stud Alcohol Drugs 2019;80(1):86–95.

34. Garcia CC, et al. Effects of age and acute moderate alcohol consumption on electrophysiological indices of attention. J Stud Alcohol Drugs 2020;81(3): 372–83.

35. Diagnostic and statistical manual 5 (DSM-5). American Psychiatric Association; 2013. Available at: http://niaaa.nih.gov/publications/brochures-and-fact-sheets/alcohol-use-disorder-comparison-between-DSM-IV-and-DSM-V. Accessed April 27,2021.

36. Smith PC, et al. Primary care validation of a single-question alcohol screening test. J Gen Intern Med 2009;24(7):783–8.

37. Available at: https://www.uspreventiveservicestaskforce.org/uspstf/recommend ation/unhealthy-alcohol-use-in-adolescents-and-adults-screening-and-behavioral-counselling-interventions#finalrecommendationstart. Accessed May 7, 2021.

38. Rockwood K, Mitnitski A. Frailty defined by accumulation of deficits and geriatric medicine defined by frailty. Clin Geriatr Med 2011;27(1):17–26r.

39. Fried LP, et al. (Cardiovascular health study collaborative research group.) frailty in older adults: evidence for a phenotype. Journals Gerontol A Biol Sci Med Sci 2001;56(3):M146–56.

40. Moos RH, et al. High-risk alcohol consumption and late-life alcohol use problems. Am J Public Health 2004;94(11):1985–91.

41. Saunders JB, et al. Development of the alcohol use disorders identification test (AUDIT): WHO collaborative project on early detection of persons with harmful alcohol consumption: II. Addiction 1993;88(6):791–804.

42. Coulton S, Dale V, Deluca P, et al. Screening for at-risk alcohol consumption in primary care: a randomized evaluation of screening approaches. Alcohol Alcohol 2017;52(3):312–7.
43. McNeely J, Adam A, Rotrosen J, et al. Comparison of methods for alcohol and drug screening in primary care clinics. JAMA Netw Open 2021;4(5):e2110721.
44. O'Mahony D. STOPP/START criteria for potentially inappropriate medications/potential prescribing omissions in older people: origin and progress. Expert Rev Clin Pharmacol 2020;13(1):15–22.
45. Bernstein E, et al. A preliminary report of knowledge translation: lessons from taking screening and brief intervention techniques from the research setting into regional systems of care. Acad Emerg Med 2009;16(11):1225–33.
46. Duru OK, Xu HY, Moore AA, et al. In: Anjani F, Smith R, Slavova S, et al, editors. Examining the impact of separate components of a multicomponent intervention designed to reduce at-risk drinking among older adults: the project SHARE. USPHTF. Accessed May 7,
47. https://www.slu.edu/medicine/internal-medicine/geriatric-medicine/aging-successfully/assessment-tools/%20Rapidhttps://www.slu.edu/medicine/internal-medicine/geriatric-medicine/aging-successfully/assessment-tools/Rapid Geriatric Assessment. Accessed May 7, 2021.
48. Bartels SJ, Coakley EH, Zubritsky C, et al. Improving access to geriatrics mental health services: a randomized trial comparing treatment engagement with integrated versus enhanced referral care for depression, anxiety and at-risk alcohol use. Am J Psychiatr 2004;16(181):1455–62.
49. Kelly S, Olanrewaju O, et al. Interventions to prevent and reduce excessive alcohol consumption in older people: a systematic review and meta-analysis. Age Aging 2018;(2):175–84.
50. Berglund KJ. Outcome in relation to drinking goals in alcohol-dependent individuals: a follow-up study 2.5 and 5 years after treatment entry. Alcohol Alcohol 2019;54(4):439–45.
51. Anton RF, et al. Combined pharmacotherapies and behavioral interventions for alcohol dependence: the COMBINE Study: a randomized controlled clinical trial. JAMA 2006;295(17):2003–17.
52. Saitz R. Medications for alcohol use disorder and predicting severe withdrawal. JAMA 2018;320(8):766–8.

Substance Misuse and the Older Offender

Samer El Hayek, MD[1], Bernadette Mdawar, MD[1], Elias Ghossoub, MD, MSc*

KEYWORDS

- Elderly • Offender • Incarceration • Prison • Judicial system • Addiction
- Substance use

KEY POINTS

- Alcohol and drug use disorders are highly prevalent among the older justice-involved population.
- Screening for substance use should be part of every comprehensive mental health assessment.
- Incorporating a biopsychosocial approach can assist with identifying risk and protective factors about substance use and determining the overall well-being of older offenders.
- Rates of recidivism may be decreased in older offenders by ensuring continuous access to integrated mental health and substance use services.

INTRODUCTION

Older adults constitute around 1% of offenders in the criminal justice system.[1] However whereas the global incarcerated population has been steadily growing over the past few years,[2] the subpopulation of older adults has been expanding at the fastest rate. In the United States, the number of state prisoners aged 55 years and older has quadrupled between 1993 and 2013, exceeding the growth rate of the total incarcerated as well as the nonincarcerated older populations.[3,4] Although aging in prisons parallels the trend in the general population,[5] the increased number of incarcerated older offenders and those serving long-term sentences in prisons explains the observed phenomena better.[4]

Defining "older offenders" has been a source of controversy. Using the "chronologic age," that is, a specific cutoff to differentiate younger from older offenders, has been commonly adopted.[6] However, whereas the age cutoff in geriatric psychiatry was set at 65 years,[7] no consensus has been reached in geriatric forensic psychiatry to date.[6]

Department of Psychiatry, American University of Beirut, P.O. Box: 11-0236, Riad El-Solh 1107 2020, Beirut, Lebanon
[1] These authors contributed equally and should be regarded as co-joint first authors.
* Corresponding author,
E-mail addresses: eg10@aub.edu.lb; elias.ghossoub@gmail.com
Twitter: @samerelhayek (S.E.H.); @bernadette_G_Md (B.M.); @EliasGhossoubMD (E.G.)

Clin Geriatr Med 38 (2022) 159–167
https://doi.org/10.1016/j.cger.2021.07.010
0749-0690/22/© 2021 Elsevier Inc. All rights reserved.

geriatric.theclinics.com

A recent systematic review that included 100 studies on the health and well-being of older offenders showed that the cutoff age ranged between 40 and 65 years and that the most selected cutoff was 50 years.[6] Key empirical evidence supporting this choice is the "accelerated aging" hypothesis that argues that incarcerated individuals' physical and mental health deteriorates 10 to 15 years earlier than the health of their non-incarcerated counterparts.[8–10] Additional empirical evidence includes shorter life expectancy, functional limitations leading to an increased reliance on the prison health care system, and earlier cognitive dysfunction.[6]

Medical and mental illnesses and substance use disorders (SUDs) are quite prevalent among older adults involved in the criminal justice system.[11] A recent systematic review found that approximately 1 of 3 incarcerated older offenders reported problematic alcohol use and approximately 1 of 4 reported drug misuse.[12] Results from the National Survey on Drug Use and Health (NSDUH) showed that, between 2015 and 2018, noninstitutionalized justice-involved adults aged 50 years or older were 3 and 8 times more likely to have a mental illness and any SUD, respectively, compared with nonjustice involved peers.[11] Furthermore, older prisoners were more than twice as likely to have any psychiatric disorder compared with older adults in the community.[13] Nevertheless, they had lower odds of anxiety disorders and cannabis and cocaine use disorders when compared with younger inmates.[14] Aging was found to have a moderating effect on the association between SUD and chronic conditions. Older inmates with a history of cannabis use disorder were at greater risk of developing psychotic disorders.[14] Similarly, cardiovascular diseases were greatly increased in older inmates with alcohol, cannabis, and injection drug use disorders; hepatitis C infection was significantly associated with cocaine and injection drug use.[14] The extent to which mental illnesses and SUD precede, co-occur with, or develop after incarceration is unclear.[15] Moreover, offending behaviors vary in their association with SUDs. We review the occurrence of different types of offenses and their relationship to drug and alcohol use among older offenders.

SUBGROUPS OF OLDER OFFENDERS

The class of older offenders encompasses 3 groups that are heterogeneous in their criminal behaviors, backgrounds, vulnerabilities, and prognosis.[16,17]

"First-time offenders" are a minority subclass composed of individuals who commit their first crime at an old age.[16,18] Compared with the other subclasses, they have a more favorable socioeconomic background and are more likely to suffer from adjustment problems during imprisonment.[16,17] Also, "first-time offenders" are less likely to have drug dependence and less likely to be convicted of drug-related offenses.[17] The second subclass of "recidivists" includes individuals who get repeatedly incarcerated at different ages due to recurrent crimes or parole violations. Recidivists commonly experience substance abuse and other chronic health problems.[16,19] Last, individuals incarcerated at a younger age but sentenced for a long period constitute the subclass of "long-term servers."[16]

Crime rates by older adults are often underestimated because crimes by this population go often undetected by the criminal justice system.[18] This fact is shown by the discrepancy between the number of self-reported offenses and the proportion of arrests among offenders.[20,21] In one study, only 2% of noninstitutionalized adults aged 65 years or older reported getting arrested after breaking the law in the past year.[20] Regardless, past-year alcohol and drug use disorders were significantly associated with increased odds of getting arrested as well as breaking the law.[20]

In the following sections, we referr to 2 main categories of offenses among older adults: "substance-related offenses," including driving under the influence (DUI) of

Table 1
US arrest rates (per 100,000) by age between 1980 and 2014 for select offenses

	Age (y)		
Offense	50–54	55–59	60–64
Drug abuse violations			
1980	30	22.6	13.1
1990	89.7	44.6	22.8
2000	173	81.9	39.1
2010	266	136	58.7
2014	290	163	72.9
Driving under the influence			
1980	587	427	271
1990	502	349	227
2000	390	266	175
2010	412	265	161
2014	356	246	149
Violent crime index offenses			
1980	74.2	47.2	30.1
1990	93.3	58.6	37.2
2000	87	55.1	35.1
2010	103	57.6	32.9
2014	107.6	62.9	33.5
Property crime index offenses			
1980	197	148	109
1990	233	171	124
2000	165	95.4	58.3
2010	260	142	74
2014	312.8	182.8	91.8

drugs or alcohol, drunkenness, drug sale/trafficking, drug manufacturing, and drug possessions, and "non-substance-related offenses" for all other offenses, including "violence-related offenses."

SUBSTANCE-RELATED OFFENSES

Data from the Bureau of Justice Statistics shows that between 1980 and 2014, arrest rates for DUI across age groups 50 to 54, 55 to 59, and 60 to 64 years have been consistently decreasing, as seen in **Table 1**.[22] In parallel, arrest rates for drug possession and drug selling/manufacturing have greatly increased.[22] However, inmates aged 50 years or older in the Iowa Department of Corrections were found to be less commonly convicted of drug-related offenses compared with their younger counterparts.[23]

Among noninstitutionalized older adults surveyed in the NSDUH between 2008 and 2014, DUI of alcohol was by far the most commonly self-reported offense (3.4%), followed by selling illegal drugs (0.7%); DUI of drugs was reported by 0.2% of the population.[20]

Studies on DUI correlates among noninstitutionalized adults aged 50 years or older invariably report greater involvement of men compared with women and the use of alcohol and illicit drugs other than marijuana.[21,24,25] Choi and colleagues[21] used NSDUH data from 2008 through 2012 to study 2 groups of older adults (aged 50–64 year and ≥65 years) with a history of past-year substance use and self-reported DUI. The investigators found that DUI of alcohol was more common than DUI of other drugs in both groups. In addition, common DUI predictors among both groups were elevated income, increased frequency of alcohol use, bingeing on alcohol in the past 30 days, marijuana use, and having a major depressive episode. Being employed, being married, having better health, and using illicit drugs other than cannabis significantly increased the odds of self-reported DUI among individuals aged 50 to 64 years; having a college degree or a lifetime arrest history significantly predicted self-reported DUI among individuals aged 65 years or older.[21] In another study based on data from NSDUH between 2012 and 2013, the investigators warned of growing safety concerns among older driving adults who use cannabis[25]; this is particularly true as self-reported DUI among older cannabis users was 7 times higher than nonusers, whereas their risk perception of cannabis was extremely low.[25]

NON-SUBSTANCE-RELATED OFFENSES

Few studies looked into alcohol and substance misuse in older adults committing non-drug-related offenses. In one retrospective cohort study of 1853 first-time offenders aged 45 years or older in Western Australia, the baseline prevalence of SUDs was 5.9% and 5.5% among violent and nonviolent offenders, respectively.[26] The investigators found that violent offenders were equally likely as nonviolent offenders to seek mental health services for SUD during the year before sentencing.[26] In a retrospective review of 210 forensic psychiatric evaluations of Swedish offenders aged 60 years or older who committed serious crimes, close to 15% of the principal diagnoses were substance abuse/dependence.[27] And in another retrospective review of trial competency or criminal responsibility evaluations of 99 adults aged 60 years or older in South Carolina, alcohol abuse/dependence was the most prevalent diagnosis (67.7%).[28] Moreover, close to 30% of these older offenders were using substances at the time of the alleged offense; this factor was not significantly associated with violent crime perpetration.[28] The discrepancies in prevalence rates of substance use across studies might be best explained by the heterogeneity of the target populations.

Research in the general population shows that substance use is associated with violent conduct. A study on cannabis use in older offenders suggested that 50- to 64-year-olds who engaged in drug selling were almost 10 times more likely to consume cannabis, whereas those who committed theft or violent attacks only had 2 and 3 times greater odds of use, respectively.[29] Alternatively, in a study using NSDUH data spanning from 2002 to 2017 to assess the characteristics of various criminal behaviors among older community-dwelling individuals, those with past-year cannabis use were found to have significantly higher odds of committing violent behaviors. Furthermore, those reporting past-year tobacco and other illicit drug use were found to have significantly higher odds of committing criminal behaviors. However, these results were not stratified by behavior subtype.[30]

TREATMENT SERVICES FOR ALCOHOL AND SUBSTANCE MISUSE IN THE OLDER OFFENDER

At present, most prison health services do not adequately integrate addiction services. Once individuals with SUDs become involved in the judicial system, they are unlikely to receive evidence-based management.[31] In addition, they have elevated rates of criminal recidivism.[32]

In a content analysis of the literature, it was found that the detection of mental health issues and access to services in older offenders are identified at different stages of the criminal justice pathway.[15] For instance, serious psychiatric disorders such as schizophrenia and neurocognitive impairment are commonly identified in the early stages. However, substance use problems are typically detected later in the criminal justice trajectory, usually during the prison intake process. Furthermore, many older prisoners frequently have difficulty accessing treatment services.[15]

Diagnostic delays in prisons are attributed to several factors, including the incomplete transmission of clinical records upon incarceration, highly stressed mental health resources within correction systems, and withholding psychiatric history due to fear of stigma and discrimination. Another hypothesis is that the prison setting itself may be stressful enough to trigger subclinical psychiatric symptoms, particularly in the setting of social isolation, lack of support, and violence.[23] One cross-sectional study found that only 67% of older offenders with an SUD diagnosis received treatment during incarceration. The most frequent treatment service was Narcotics Anonymous. Formal programs, one-on-one counseling, and pharmacologic management were less commonly reported.[33] These results emphasize the importance of timely diagnosis, particularly in special populations such as older offenders, to ensure receipt of adequate services and optimize health care outcomes throughout the imprisonment period. Case in point, one recent systematic review found that prisoners with opioid use disorder who were treated with opioid agonist treatment during their incarceration were more likely to adhere to substance use treatment and were less likely to relapse into illicit opioid use or to be reincarcerated.[34]

Along the same lines, when looking into older offenders with SUDs and comorbid pain, adequate management can be impeded by physicians' fear of misuse, diversion of medication, or overdosing. As a result, offenders' quality of life can be significantly altered.[35] Developing a tailored approach for the assessment and management of pain and other medical conditions in this subgroup is recommended.

More studies looked into the management of substance misuse services in older offenders postincarceration. One cross-sectional study investigated factors associated with illicit substance use after release from incarceration.[33] Variables significantly associated with higher postrelease illicit substance use were male gender, housing with family or friends, a longer period between release and the first medical encounter, and having an SUD diagnosis. Alternatively, a greater period of incarceration and being on parole were associated with lower odds of postrelease illicit substance use.[33]

When looking into factors that can help achieve sobriety and prevent relapse, a qualitative study of 15 elderly inmates released from prison noted age as central to the process.[36] This observation was closely associated with a growing awareness of their mortality. Prison time also allowed inmates to reflect upon the lives they led before incarceration and to plan for a different path after release, based on newly identified goals and values incompatible with drug use. In addition, the period of forced detoxification after initial incarceration and the prolonged period of sobriety throughout the prison stay acted as a catalyst for this process.[36] These results are concordant with clinical data revealing that older age[37] and an involuntary period of sobriety[38,39] may set individuals with SUDs on a new trajectory.

When looking into challenges that can trigger relapse following prison release older offenders pinpoint several themes, including medical issues and social challenges such as discrimination, stigma, limited familial support, and prior associations with negative peers. Other noted challenges encompass financial difficulties, particularly in getting employed and having housing, and psychological difficulties with older offenders being highly susceptible to triggers.[40] Along the same lines, Western and colleagues (2015)[41] found that released older prisoners, particularly those with SUDs, were the most socially disconnected and materially disadvantaged (insecurely housed and less likely to be employed).

Despite these challenges, older former prisoners are less likely to recidivate than their younger counterparts and more likely to progress through treatment, complete it, commit to conventional goals, and refrain from relapse.[42,43] Chamberlain and colleagues (2018)[33] noted that among released older prisoners who had a history of SUD, only one-quarter reported illicit substance use following release.

Overall, data are limited about the types of monitoring practices that are most effective after release. Close supervision is considered best practice.[44] If participants' parole monitoring included urine drug testing, this may effectively discourage illicit substance use.[33] Also, while it is important to provide material resources for this vulnerable subgroup, it is equally necessary for community organizations to help repair and provide prosocial bonds.

SUMMARY

Alcohol and drug use disorders are highly prevalent among the older justice-involved population. Screening for substance use should be part of every comprehensive mental health assessment. Many studies found that completing such an assessment significantly increases the referral of older offenders to mental health services, whether court-mandated or in the prison setting.[15] Incorporating a biopsychosocial approach can also assist with identifying risk and protective factors about substance use and determining the overall mental and medical well-being of older offenders.[15] Such an approach requires an interprofessional team that includes mental health professionals, medical practitioners, and social services, among others.

Other relevant areas for intervention include postincarceration aftercare for substance use. Rates of recidivism may be decreased in older offenders by ensuring continuous access to integrated mental health and substance use services, not only during incarceration but also after release from custody. A community-wide strategy that takes into consideration the role of social determinants must be adopted when treating SUDs in older offenders. These services should be particularly targeted to those with the greatest risk factors and treatment needs.

CLINICS CARE POINTS

- "Older offenders," primarily defined as individuals aged 50 years and older who are involved in the criminal justice system, have high rates of alcohol and drug misuse as well as other chronic mental and medical conditions.

- Low rates of substance-related offenses have been described in the literature, of which DUI of alcohol and/or drugs has been the most common.

- Preliminary data show that older offenders with violence-related offenses tend to have lower proportions of substance misuse compared with those with substance-related offenses.

- The detection of substance misuse and referral to relevant treatment services typically occur later in the criminal justice pathways for older offenders.

- Older former prisoners are less likely to recidivate and more likely to progress through substance use treatment compared with their younger peers.
- There is a need for timely diagnosis and treatment of substance misuse in older offenders while adopting a biopsychosocial model and ensuring close follow-up in the community after release.

DISCLOSURE

The authors have nothing to disclose.

REFERENCES

1. Zurek O, Stanton L, Kohn R. Sociopathy, antisocial personality, and directed aggression in the geriatric population. In: Holzer JC, Kohn R, Ellison JM, et al, editors. Geriatric forensic psychiatry: principles and practice. New York, NY: Oxford University Press; 2018. p. 191–7.
2. Walmsley R. World prison population list. 12th edition. London, UK: Institute for Criminal Policy Research; 2018. Available at: https://www.prisonstudies.org/research-publications?shs_term_node_tid_depth=27. Accessed May 23, 2021.
3. Williams BA, Goodwin JS, Baillargeon J, et al. Addressing the aging crisis in U.S. criminal justice health care. J Am Geriatr Soc 2012;60(6):1150–6.
4. Carson EA, Sabol WJ. Aging of the state prison population. May report (NCJ 248766). Washington, DC: Bureau of Justice Statistics, US Department of Justice; 2016.
5. United Nations, Department of Economic and Social Affairs, Population Division. World population ageing 2019 (ST/ESA/SER.A/444). 2020. Available at: https://www.un-ilibrary.org/content/books/9789210045544. Accessed May 23, 2021.
6. Merkt H, Haesen S, Meyer L, et al. Defining an age cut-off for older offenders: a systematic review of literature. Int J Prison Health 2020;16(2):95–116.
7. World Health Organization. Division of mental health and prevention of substance abuse & world psychiatric association. Psychiatry of the elderly: a consensus statement. World health organization. 1996. Available at: https://apps.who.int/iris/handle/10665/63623. Accessed May 23, 2021.
8. Loeb SJ, Steffensmeier D, Lawrence F. Comparing incarcerated and community-dwelling older men's health. West J Nurs Res 2007;30(2):234–49.
9. Fazel S, Hope T, O'Donnell I, et al. Health of elderly male prisoners: worse than the general population, worse than younger prisoners. Age Ageing 2001;30(5):403–7.
10. Combalbert N, Pennequin V, Ferrand C, et al. Mental disorders and cognitive impairment in ageing offenders. J Forensic Psychiatry Psychol 2016;27(6):853–66.
11. Han BH, Williams BA, Palamar JJ. Medical multimorbidity, mental illness, and substance use disorder among middle-aged and older justice-involved adults in the USA, 2015-2018. J Gen Intern Med 2020;36(5):1258–63.
12. Solares C, Dobrosavljevic M, Larsson H, et al. The mental and physical health of older offenders: a systematic review and meta-analysis. Neurosci Biobehav Rev 2020;118:440–50.
13. Di Lorito C, Völlm B, Dening T. Psychiatric disorders among older prisoners: a systematic review and comparison study against older people in the community. Aging Ment Health 2018;22(1):1–10.

14. Gates ML, Staples-Horne M, Walker V, et al. Substance use disorders and related health problems in an aging offender population. J Health Care Poor Underserved 2017;28(2s):132–54.

15. Maschi T, Dasarathy D. Aging with mental disorders in the criminal justice system: a content analysis of the empirical literature. Int J Offender Ther Comp Criminol 2019;63(12):2103–37.

16. Morton JB. An administrative overview of the older inmate. Washington, DC: US Department of Justice, National Institute of Corrections; 1992.

17. DeLisi M, Tahja KN, Drury AJ, et al. De novo advanced adult-onset offending: new evidence from a population of federal correctional clients. J Forensic Sci 2018; 63(1):172–7.

18. Kirk DS. Examining the divergence across self-report and official data sources on inferences about the adolescent life-course of crime. J Quant Criminol 2006; 22(2):107–29.

19. Neeley CL, Addison L, Craig-Moreland D. Addressing the needs of elderly offenders. Correct Today 1997;59(5):120–3.

20. Ghossoub E, Khoury R. Prevalence and correlates of criminal behavior among the non-institutionalized elderly: results from the national Survey on drug use and health. J Geriatr Psychiatry Neurol 2018;31(4):211–22.

21. Choi NG, DiNitto DM, Marti CN. Risk factors for self-reported driving under the influence of alcohol and/or illicit drugs among older adults. Gerontologist 2016; 56(2):282–91.

22. Snyder HN, Cooper AD, Mulako-Wangota J. USA Arrest rates by age between 1980 and 2014 for select offenses. Generated using the arrest data analysis tool. 2021. Available at: www.bjs.gov. Accessed on: May 23, 2021.

23. Al-Rousan T, Rubenstein L, Sieleni B, et al. Inside the nation's largest mental health institution: a prevalence study in a state prison system. BMC Public Health 2017;17(1):1–9.

24. Malek-Ahmadi M. Age-associated alcohol and driver risk differences in older adult DUI offenders. J Appl Gerontol 2017;36(4):499–507.

25. Choi NG, DiNitto DM, Marti CN. Older adults driving under the influence: associations with marijuana use, marijuana use disorder, and risk perceptions. J Appl Gerontol 2019;38(12):1687–707.

26. Sodhi-Berry N, Knuiman M, Alan J, et al. Pre- and post-sentence mental health service use by a population cohort of older offenders (≥45 years) in Western Australia. Soc Psychiatry Psychiatr Epidemiol 2015;50(7):1097–110.

27. Fazel S, Grann M. Older criminals: a descriptive study of psychiatrically examined offenders in Sweden. Int J Geriatr Psychiatry 2002;17(10):907–13.

28. Lewis CF, Fields C, Rainey E. A study of geriatric forensic evaluees: who are the violent elderly? J Am Acad Psychiatry Law 2006;34(3):324–32.

29. Salas-Wright CP, Vaughn MG, Cummings-Vaughn LA, et al. Trends and correlates of marijuana use among late middle-aged and older adults in the United States, 2002-2014. Drug Alcohol Depend 2017;171:97–106.

30. Holzer KJ, AbiNader MA, Vaughn MG, et al. Crime and violence in older adults: findings from the 2002 to 2017 National Survey on Drug Use and Health. J Interpers Violence 2020. 886260520913652.

31. Wakeman SE, Rich JD. Addiction treatment within U.S. Correctional facilities: Bridging the gap between current practice and evidence-based care. J Addict Dis 2015;34(2–3):220–5.

32. Håkansson A, Berglund M. Risk factors for criminal recidivism - a prospective follow-up study in prisoners with substance abuse. BMC Psychiatry 2012;12:111.

33. Chamberlain A, Nyamu S, Aminawung J, et al. Illicit substance use after release from prison among formerly incarcerated primary care patients: a cross-sectional study. Addict Sci Clin Pract 2019;14(1):7.

34. Malta M, Varatharajan T, Russell C, et al. Opioid-related treatment, interventions, and outcomes among incarcerated persons: a systematic review. PLoS Med 2019;16(12):e1003002.

35. Haesen S, Merkt H, Imber A, et al. Substance use and other mental health disorders among older prisoners. Int J Law Psychiatry 2019;62:20–31.

36. Wyse JJ. Older former prisoners' pathways to sobriety. Alcohol Treat Q 2018; 36(1):32–53.

37. Best DW, Ghufran S, Day E, et al. Breaking the habit: a retrospective analysis of desistance factors among formerly problematic heroin users. Drug Alcohol Rev 2008;27(6):619–24.

38. Cepeda A, Nowotny KM, Valdez A. Trajectories of aging long-term Mexican American heroin injectors: the "maturing out" paradox. J Aging Health 2016; 28(1):19–39.

39. Levy JA, Anderson T. The drug career of the older injector. Addict Res Theor 2005;13(3):245–58.

40. SACA. Reintegration needs and challenges faced by elderly ex-offenders in Singapore. Singapore: Singapore After-Care Association; 2018.

41. Western B, Braga AA, Davis J, et al. Stress and hardship after prison. AJS 2015; 120(5):1512–47.

42. Gordon MS, Kinlock TW, Couvillion KA, et al. A Randomized clinical trial of methadone maintenance for prisoners: prediction of treatment entry and completion in prison. J Offender Rehabil 2012;51(4):222–38.

43. Zanis DA, Coviello DM, Lloyd JJ, et al. Predictors of drug treatment completion among parole violators. J Psychoactive Drugs 2009;41(2):173–80.

44. Marlowe DB. Integrating substance abuse treatment and criminal justice supervision. Sci Pract Perspect 2003;2(1):4–14.

Prevention Strategies of Alcohol and Substance Use Disorders in Older Adults

Samer El Hayek, MD[a], Luna Geagea, MD[a], Hussein El Bourji, BS[b],
Tamara Kadi, BA[b], Farid Talih, MD[a],*

KEYWORDS

- Substance use disorder • Addiction • Older adults • Prevention • Screening
- Assessment

INTRODUCTION

Substance use is one of the fastest-growing health problems among older adults in the United States, with nearly 1 million adults aged 65 years and older living with a substance use disorder (SUD).[1] This situation is partially attributed to the aging baby boomer generation; this population has had more exposure to alcohol, tobacco, and drugs from a younger age than any preceding generation and has been affected by shifting social attitudes regarding substances.[2,3] With the first of the baby boomer generation turning 65 in 2011, the US Census Bureau estimated that, by 2029, more than 20% of the population will be 65 years and older, causing a "gray tsunami" demographic shift.[4] Despite the increase in the number of older adults with SUDs, addiction is often undetected and undertreated in this population.[3]

According to the *Diagnostic and Statistical Manual of Mental Disorders* (Fifth Edition), the diagnosis of SUDs requires a pattern of use that causes clinically significant functional impairment. Strict use of these criteria may be problematic in older adults and requires to be individualized to identify at-risk individuals whose substance use is excessive and harmful to their physical and mental health.[5]

SUDs may be difficult to recognize in older adults owing to associated medical comorbidity, comorbid psychiatric illness, neurocognitive decline, and functional impairment associated with aging. Substance use can also complicate the course and management of existing medical problems.[6,7] Older adults with SUDs have higher hospitalization rates and acute health care costs, compared with the general population.[8]

Given the negative impacts of SUDs on the aging population, screening and prevention of substance use are critical to improve quality of life and address the public health impact of addiction in older adults.

[a] Department of Psychiatry, American University of Beirut, P.O. Box: 11-0236, Riad El-Solh 1107 2020, Beirut, Lebanon; [b] American University of Beirut, Beirut, Lebanon
* Corresponding author.
E-mail address: Ft10@aub.edu.lb
Twitter: @samerelhayek (S.E.H.); @faridtalih (F.T.)

Clin Geriatr Med 38 (2022) 169–179
https://doi.org/10.1016/j.cger.2021.07.011
0749-0690/22/© 2021 Elsevier Inc. All rights reserved.

geriatric.theclinics.com

DISCUSSION
Impact of Substance Use on Older Adults

Alcohol
Alcohol is the most commonly used substance in older adults, with rates steadily increasing over the past years.[9,10] According to the 2018 National Survey on Drug Use and Health (NSDUH), over the past month, around one-tenth and one-fortieth of older adults engaged in binge drinking and heavy drinking, respectively. In addition, 1.6% of adults were diagnosed with alcohol use disorder.[1] Compared with other age groups, increases in alcohol use disorder and high-risk drinking were the greatest for older adults.[11]

Even though moderate alcohol consumption can have beneficial health outcomes, severe and heavy drinking in older adults has been associated with increased emergency visits and hospitalizations.[11,12] Alcohol use was also found to increase mortality in a dose-dependent fashion in older adults; the more drinks one has, the higher the risk.[13,14] Hence, there is a need to design specific prevention strategies that target this portion of the population.

Alcohol affects older individuals differently than their younger counterparts; this can be attributed to the natural physiologic changes that accompany aging.[15] These effects include a decrease in lean body mass and total body water, reduced liver function, decline in the metabolism of alcohol, and increase in blood-brain permeability and neuronal sensitivity to alcohol.[15] As such, for the same amount of alcohol consumed, older adults will experience a higher blood alcohol concentration compared with young individuals and will be at greater risk for developing unfavorable outcomes.[15] Older women are also more sensitive than men to the effects of alcohol.[16]

Acutely, drinking can impair one's judgment, coordination, and reaction putting them at an increased risk for falls, fractures, injuries, and even motor accidents; this is particularly concerning for older adults who might have a preexisting neurocognitive impairment, gait/balance problems, and decreased bone density.[16] In the long term, as older adults tend to have chronic medical problems such as cardiovascular disorders, alcohol can potentially exacerbate these conditions. Alcohol can also increase the risk of cirrhosis and impair the immune system, affecting one's ability to fight infections.[16] Furthermore, drinking can accelerate the cognitive deterioration that often accompanies aging; alcohol may also lead to confusion and forgetfulness, which is sometimes misdiagnosed as dementia.[16] Excessive alcohol use, defined as 21 or more drinks/wk, is by itself a modifiable risk factor of dementia; eliminating use starting midlife reduces dementia prevalence by 1%.[17]

Moreover, alcohol can interfere with the absorption, distribution, and metabolism of medications. This interference can lead to hazardous outcomes, especially in older adults who have high levels of polypharmacy.[18] Alcohol-drug interactions can cause lightheadedness, blood pressure fluctuations, gouty flares, and oversedation.[16] In addition, alcohol increases the risk of several malignancies and exacerbates chronic conditions such as diabetes and depression.[18]

Tobacco
Around 8.2% of older adults are smokers.[19] Although this rate is lower than that in younger adults, it remains highly associated with adverse health outcomes. Smoking and increased nicotine dependence were shown to be correlated with lower quality of life among this population.[20] Older adults who smoke have an increased risk of becoming frail and sustaining fractures.[21] Smoking in this age group is also associated with health risks different from those in younger counterparts. For younger smokers,

cardiovascular disease remains the major contributor to smoking-related mortality. Alternatively, a shift toward lung cancer and chronic obstructive pulmonary disease is observed among older smokers.[22]

Although about 300,000 smoking-related deaths occur each year among individuals aged 65 years and older, the risk diminishes in older adults who quit smoking.[19] A typical smoker who quits after the age of 65 years could add 2 to 3 years to their life expectancy. In addition, within a year of quitting, most former smokers reduce their risk of coronary heart disease by half.[19] Smoking cessation interventions implemented in midlife and late life also contribute to a 5% estimated risk reduction of dementia prevalence in older adults.[23]

Smoking cessation is the most effective tool to decrease smoking-related morbidity and mortality across all ages, even though its advantages are partially limited among older adults and may manifest at a slower pace. Older smokers are less likely to attempt, but more likely to succeed in quitting smoking.[22]

Cannabis
Cannabis is the most used substance in older adults following alcohol and tobacco.[1] Past-year cannabis use in this population sharply increased from only 0.15% in 2002 to 4.2% in 2018.[24] This increase in cannabis use is likely related to more permissive societal attitudes for recreational and medicinal uses of marijuana. Legalization across many states in the United States and the emergence of novel evidence for cannabis medicinal benefits also contribute to the increasing consumption across all age groups.[25,26]

The main indications for medical use of cannabis are weight loss, depression, anxiety, sleep disturbances, and chronic pain. These conditions are common among older adults, making cannabis use frequent in this age group.[26,27] The use of cannabis can, however, be harmful, especially in older adults,[27,28] because aging increases the effects of cannabis by the same physiologic mechanisms that increase those of alcohol.[15] While being treated with cannabis several older adults report acute adverse effects, most commonly dizziness, fatigue, and sleepiness.[27] Cannabis use can also cause paradoxic anxiety, tachycardia, and hypertension. More importantly, the risk of having a heart attack increases 4-fold following an hour of cannabis smoking.[29] In addition, cannabis use has been linked to the occurrence of cerebrovascular events such as strokes, a risk typically more prominent with aging.[30] Cannabis can also impair both short- and long-term memory,[29,31] and prolonged use has been linked to cognitive impairment and slower processing speed,[32] effects that can be more pronounced in older adults. Last, both current and former users of cannabis are at higher risk of developing a mental disorder when compared with nonusers.[33] Furthermore, the prevalence of past-year substance use is typically greater in cannabis users compared with nonusers,[1] suggesting that the harmful effects of cannabis in older adults might be partially mediated by other substances.

Prescription medications
Several studies looked into the prevalence of prescription medication misuse among older adults; prevalence rates ranged from 1% to 26%.[34] One study found that 7.7% of US adults aged 50 years and older with past-year use of prescription medication misused it.[35] Surprisingly, older adults are prescribed opioids and benzodiazepines at comparatively higher rates than other age cohorts, despite clinical recommendations that advise against this because of their harmful side effects in this age group.[36] According to the 2018 NSDUH, about 1.6 million adults aged 26 years or older misused opioids in the past year; adults aged 50 years and older were least likely to

misuse opioids.[1] Despite these findings, the NSDUH data suggest that opioid misuse is increasing among older adults. From 1995 to 2010, opioids prescribed for older adults during regular office visits increased by a factor of 9.[37] Between 2013 and 2015, the proportion of people in that age group seeking treatment of opioid use disorder increased nearly 54%, whereas the proportion of older adults using heroin more than doubled.[38]

Older adults are vulnerable to misusing prescription medications because they are more likely to be prescribed medications with misuse prospects compared with younger individuals. These medications are typically given for the management of conditions common in older adults, such as chronic pain, sleep, and anxiety disorders. Older adults are also at risk for adverse effects due to their increased fragility, reduced metabolism, and slower elimination of drugs[34]; this heightens the risk of drug-drug interactions, adverse effects, and organ damage.[35]

Prevention Strategies

Older adults with SUDs are frequently treated for both addiction and chronic health problems in an uncoordinated manner. The presence of barriers for the identification of SUDs in older adults can further impair management (**Table 1**).[5] Clinicians should be aware of the complex interaction between aging, chronic medical conditions, and substance misuse to efficiently implement a geriatric-focused approach for the management of SUDs. Many of the fundamentals of harm reduction and preventative medicine for chronic diseases intersect, such as shared decision making and patient-centered care. Most models that have integrated these principles emphasize substance use outcomes rather than health-related ones; this is where the gap in research and clinical work lies.[2,39,40]

When considering preventative measures, clinicians should initially target substances that are relatively common in older adults, particularly alcohol and nicotine. Alcohol misuse can be reduced if proper prevention and early intervention approaches are taken, especially those targeting risk and protective factors corresponding to this population. One such program is the aging services network, which delivers social and supportive aid to older adults.[41] Other population-based prevention strategies include health education programs about unsafe drinking rituals and methods to restrict

Table 1	
Barriers to the identification of SUDs in older adults	
	Barriers
Physician-related	Stereotypes about older adults, stereotypes about addiction, lack of knowledge about treatment[5]
Patient-related	Shame, guilt, stigma, denial[5]
Diagnostic factors	Presence of age-related changes or comorbid conditions that may obscure or be used to explain symptoms of SUDs, lower applicability of DSM-V criteria in older adults (ie, age group more susceptible to smaller amounts of substances leading to lower tolerance and subtle withdrawal, different role obligations compared with younger adults, and engagement in fewer activities regardless of SUDs)[5]

Abbreviation: DSM-5, Diagnostic and Statistical Manual of Mental Disorders (Fifth Edition).

excessive alcohol consumption. Other strategies include preventive visits with the primary care physician, screening, and brief interventions in the primary care setting. Brief medical advice by a family physician has been shown to decrease alcohol use in older adults and alleviate potential adverse health outcomes.[42]

In terms of tobacco prevention in older adults, the field remains in its infancy. Some effective programs have been proved to be successful among this age group, including customized brief interventions which increase 1-year quit rates by more than 2-fold.[43] Community-based interventions also play an important role, with effective interventions such as increasing tobacco prices, comprehensive smoke-free policies, educational campaigns, and barrier-free access to tobacco cessation counseling and medications.[19] As clinicians typically advise older adults to quit smoking they fail to provide evidence-based strategies; physicians should be more proactive in offering or referring to evidence-based cessation treatments.[44]

In light of the opioid epidemic, prudent prescribing practices can prevent prescription drug misuse. Clinicians should be aware of a patient's history of SUDs and try to avoid prescribing medications that increase the risk for misuse or relapse. Prescription drug monitoring programs and online training programs for opiate prescribing and management of chronic pain are important resources to ensure safe prescribing.[45]

Another important target of focus is polypharmacy, a common phenomenon among older adults, particularly those with chronic medical problems.[46] Polypharmacy can increase the likelihood of adverse drug reactions, falls, and hospitalizations in older adults; it can also worsen the medical and psychological repercussions of any underlying SUD. To avoid such drawbacks, the prevention of polypharmacy is necessary and possible. For instance, one study estimated that around 1 in 5 drugs prescribed to older adults can be stopped or substituted with a safer option.[47] Therefore, clinicians must regularly discuss multiple drug usage with their patients and enquire about the intake of over-the-counter medications and herbal or vitamin supplements. The implementation of prescription drug monitoring programs remains of utmost importance.[46]

Clinical Assessment

When assessing SUDs in older adults, some general considerations apply. The assessment should include a respectful, nonstigmatizing, and nonconfrontational attitude. Older adults are more likely to offer information about potentially stigmatizing behaviors if they believe that the clinician is genuinely interested in their well-being. Clinicians should use medically accurate terms of "substance use disorder" and "unhealthy use" while refraining from discriminatory words such as "abuser" or "addict." Discussions of SUDs should always occur in the context of an overall assessment. Special considerations are recommended when treating particularly vulnerable subgroups, such as the elderly lesbian, gay, bisexual, transgender, and questioning (LGBTQ) population.[48] An inclusive and nonjudgmental approach is essential for successful treatment programs.

Moreover, clinicians should keep in mind relevant risk factors[5,49] and potential indicators for SUDs (**Table 2**).[5] The focus should be on the facts of substance use, with direct questions about nicotine, alcohol, prescription medication, and illicit drug use.

Uniform screening and detailed systematic history taking should be the norm when assessing older adults for SUDs. This approach often reduces stigma by normalizing the screening behavior for the patient.[3,5]

Table 2
Risk factors and indicators of substance use disorders in older adults

	Risk Factors	Indicators
Physical health	Chronic physical illness, chronic pain conditions, physical disability, reduced cognition[5]	Falls, bruises, burns, poor nutrition, poor hygiene, incontinence, headaches, dizziness, sensory deficits, memory loss, blackouts, disorientation, reduced cognition, idiopathic seizures[5]
Mental health	Comorbid psychiatric disorders (including posttraumatic stress disorder and adverse childhood experiences), sleep disorders[5]	Anxiety, depression, mood swings, sleep disturbances, paranoia, delusions[5]
Medications	Polypharmacy[5]	Running out of medication early, borrowing from others, increased tolerance, or unusual response to medications[5]
Social factors	Limited social support, social isolation, grief and bereavement, unexpected or forced retirement, changes in living situation[5]	Family problems, financial problems, legal problems, social isolation[5]

Screening and Intervention

Screening, brief intervention, and referral to treatment (SBIRT) for SUDs is a US nationwide, evidence-based, public health strategy to treat addiction.[50] This approach applies to older adults. Building on it, several screening instruments are available, with few designed specifically for older adults, which can help identify underlying SUDs and initiate a brief intervention or referral, as deemed necessary (**Table 3**).[2,51–55]

In cases of positive screening, several effective brief interventions centered on educating about harm and enhancing motivation for change can occur in the primary care setting. Such interventions incorporate patient feedback, brief advice, and motivational interviewing. These interventions vary in duration from 10 to 15 minutes to multiple extended sessions and seem to be highly effective in older adults.[3,5] Motivational interviewing, in particular, is a communication method that uses client-centered counseling to elicit motivation and reduce ambivalence for behavior change; it seeks to strengthen the client's motivations for change and follows a concrete plan of action in an evocative and collaborative setting. This technique was found useful for older adults within the primary care setting.[56,57]

Alternatively, those with more severe SUDs tend to require intensive treatments. These individuals should be referred to specialized professionals and advanced treatment services. Group treatments, including self-help groups, are also typically recommended for older adults. The treatment plan should always be individualized and flexible according to the specific needs of the patient.[3,5]

Table 3
Screening tools for substance use disorders in the general population and older adults

Substance	Tool	Description
Polysubstance	SUBS[53]	The Substance Use Brief Screen is a self-administered brief screener for tobacco, alcohol, and drug use validated in primary care settings. Screening positive would lead to further screening
	ASSIST[51,52]	The Alcohol, Smoking, and Substance Involvement Screening Test covers all psychoactive substances in primary care settings. This test determines a risk score for each substance. The score for each substance falls into a "lower-," "moderate-," or "high"-risk category, which determines the most appropriate intervention for that level of use ("no treatment," "brief intervention," or "referral to specialist assessment and treatment," respectively)
Alcohol	CAGE[2,51,52] CAGE-AID[2,53]	The acronym CAGE comes from the wording of the 4 questions asked; it is used in primary care to detect lifetime alcohol use disorders, with a sensitivity of 86% and specificity of 78%. CAGE-AID is the CAGE Adapted to Include Drug use
	AUDIT[2,51,52,55] AUDIT-5[53] AUDIT-C[51,52]	The Alcohol Use Disorders Identification Test is a 10-item survey that assesses alcohol consumption, drinking behaviors, and alcohol-related problems in the past year. This test has high specificity (91%) but low sensitivity (33%) in older adults. AUDIT-5 and AUDIT-C are 5- and 3-item shorter versions for primary care settings, respectively
	ARPS[a53] shARPS[a53]	The Alcohol-Related Problems Survey (60-item instrument) and the Short ARPS (32-item instrument) identify older persons whose use of alcohol alone or in combination with their comorbidities, medications, symptoms, and functional status may be causing them harm or placing them at risk for harm
	MAST-G[a51,52] SMAST-G[a52]	The Michigan Alcohol Screening Test-Geriatric Version is a 25-item instrument used if patients report regular alcohol use. Two or more "yes" responses suggest an alcohol problem. SMAST-G is a shorter 13-item version with a sensitivity of 93.9% and a specificity of 78.1%
	CARET[a2,53]	The 27-item Comorbidity-Alcohol Risk Evaluation Tool identifies older adults with specific health behaviors and risks that place them at increased risk for harm from alcohol. This tool has a sensitivity of 92% and a specificity of 51%
Nicotine	FTND[51,52] HIS[53]	The Fagerstrom test for nicotine dependence is a 10-item self-report instrument. A score of ≥3 is customarily suggestive of nicotine dependence. The Heavy Smoking Index is a briefer measure that includes only 2 FTND items. A high HSI of ≥4 is a good and briefer alternative for detecting high nicotine dependence
	mCEQ[53]	The modified Cigarette Evaluation Questionnaire is a 5-item self-report instrument that assesses the reinforcing effects of smoking cigarettes from a smoker's perspective
	CDS-12[54] CDS-5[54]	The 12-item Cigarette Dependence Scale assesses dependence with an emphasis on compulsion to smoke,

(continued on next page)

Table 3 *(continued)*		
Substance	**Tool**	**Description**
		withdrawal, loss of control, time allocation, neglect of other activities, and persistence despite harm. CDS-5 is a shorter version
Opioids	SOAPP[53]	The Screener and Opioid Assessment for Patients in Pain is a self-report measure designed to assess the appropriateness of long-term opioid therapy for patients with chronic pain. A score of ≥ 7 indicates an increased risk of abuse
	COMM[53]	The Current Opioid Misuse Measure is a 17-item self-report instrument designed to identify patients with chronic pain taking opioids who have indicators of current aberrant drug-related behaviors. A score of ≥ 9 indicates medication misuse and increased risk of abuse
	DAST[51,52]	The Drug Abuse Screening Test is a 28-item self-report instrument that consists of items that parallel those of the MAST but screen for abuse of drugs other than alcohol. Cutoff scores of 6 through 11 are considered to be optimal for screening for SUDs

[a] Screening tool specific for older adults.[a]

SUMMARY

The number of older adults who engage in unhealthy substance use has been increasing. It is important to recognize the unique challenges in the identification, prevention, and screening of SUDs in this age group. Appropriate screening and the implementation of targeted prevention and intervention strategies can be key in improving insight, reducing stigma, and improving outcomes and overall quality of life in this vulnerable population.

CLINICS CARE POINTS

- Substance use is one of the fastest-growing health problems among older adults in the United States. Alcohol, nicotine, and cannabis are the most commonly misused substances in this age group.

- Clinicians should be aware of the complex interaction between addiction, chronic medical problems, aging, and polypharmacy.

- Clinical assessment should include a respectful and nonstigmatizing attitude, with screening, brief intervention, and referral to treatment when indicated.

DISCLOSURE

The authors have nothing to disclose.

REFERENCES

1. Detailed tables. Rockville, MD: Center for Behavioral Health Statistics and Quality, Substance Abuse and Mental Health Services Administration.: Substance Abuse and Mental Health Services Administration; 2019.

2. Han BH, Moore AA. Prevention and screening of unhealthy substance use by older adults. Clin Geriatr Med 2018;34(1):117–29.

3. Kuerbis A. Substance use among older adults: an update on prevalence, etiology, assessment, and intervention. Gerontology 2020;66(3):249–58.

4. 2020 census will help policymakers prepare for the incoming wave of aging boomers. 2019. Available at: https://www.census.gov/library/stories/2019/12/by-2030-all-baby-boomers-will-be-age-65-or-older.html. Accessed May 16, 2021.

5. Kuerbis A, Sacco P, Blazer DG, et al. Substance abuse among older adults. Clin Geriatr Med 2014;30(3):629–54.

6. Gossop M, Moos R. Substance misuse among older adults: a neglected but treatable problem. Addiction 2008;103(3):347–8.

7. Seim L, Vijapura P, Pagali S, et al. Common substance use disorders in older adults. Hosp Pract 2020;48(sup1):48–55.

8. Gryczynski J, Schwartz RP, O'Grady KE, et al. Understanding patterns of high-cost health care use across different substance user groups. Health Aff (Millwood) 2016;35(1):12–9.

9. Grant BF, Chou SP, Saha TD, et al. Prevalence of 12-month alcohol use, high-risk drinking, and dsm-iv alcohol use disorder in the United States, 2001-2002 to 2012-2013: Results from the national epidemiologic survey on alcohol and related conditions. JAMA Psychiatry 2017;74(9):911–23.

10. Moore AA, Karno MP, Grella CE, et al. Alcohol, tobacco, and nonmedical drug use in older U.S. adults: data from the 2001/02 national epidemiologic survey of alcohol and related conditions. J Am Geriatr Soc 2009;57(12):2275–81.

11. White AM, Castle IP, Hingson RW, et al. Using death certificates to explore changes in alcohol-related mortality in the United States, 1999 to 2017. Alcohol Clin Exp Res 2020;44(1):178–87.

12. Mattson M, Lipari RN, Hays C, et al. A day in the life of older adults: Substance use facts. In: The CBHSQ report. Rockville, MD: Center for behavioral health Statistics and quality, substance Abuse and mental health services Administration; 2017.

13. Mostofsky E, Mukamal KJ, Giovannucci EL, et al. Key findings on alcohol consumption and a variety of health outcomes from the nurses' health study. Am J Public Health 2016;106(9):1586–91.

14. O'Keefe EL, DiNicolantonio JJ, O'Keefe JH, et al. Alcohol and cv health: Jekyll and hyde j-curves. Prog Cardiovasc Dis 2018;61(1):68–75.

15. Kennedy GJ, Efremova I, Frazier A, et al. The emerging problems of alcohol and substance abuse in late life. J Soc Distress Homeless 1999;8(4):227–39.

16. NIH. Facts about aging and alcohol. Available at: https://www.nia.nih.gov/health/facts-about-aging-and-alcohol. Accessed May 16, 2021.

17. Livingston G, Huntley J, Sommerlad A, et al. Dementia prevention, intervention, and care: 2020 report of the lancet commission. Lancet 2020; 396(10248):413–46.

18. Moore AA, Whiteman EJ, Ward KT. Risks of combined alcohol/medication use in older adults. Am J Geriatr Pharmacother 2007;5(1):64–74.

19. CDC. Smoking and tobacco use: data and statistics. 2021. Available at: https://www.cdc.gov/tobacco/data_statistics/index.htm?s_cid=osh-stu-home-nav-005. Accessed May 16, 2021.

20. Viana DA, Andrade FCD, Martins LC, et al. Differences in quality of life among older adults in Brazil according to smoking status and nicotine dependence. Health Qual Life Outcomes 2019;17(1):1.

21. Kojima G, Iliffe S, Jivraj S, et al. Does current smoking predict future frailty? The English longitudinal study of ageing. Age and Ageing. 2018;47(1):126–31.

22. Burns DM. Cigarette smoking among the elderly: disease consequences and the benefits of cessation. Am J Health Promot 2000;14(6):357–61.

23. Livingston G, Sommerlad A, Orgeta V, et al. Dementia prevention, intervention, and care. Lancet 2017;390(10113):2673–734.

24. Han BH, Palamar JJ. Trends in cannabis use among older adults in the United States, 2015-2018. JAMA Intern Med 2020;180(4):609–11.

25. Daniller A. Two-thirds of americans support marijuana legalization. 2019. Available at: https://www.pewresearch.org/fact-tank/2019/11/14/americans-support-marijuana-legalization/. Accessed May 16, 2021.

26. Walsh Z, Callaway R, Belle-Isle L, et al. Cannabis for therapeutic purposes: patient characteristics, access, and reasons for use. Int J Drug Policy. 2013; 24(6):511–6.

27. Abuhasira R, Ron A, Sikorin I, et al. Medical cannabis for older patients-treatment protocol and initial results. J Clin Med 2019;8(11):1819.

28. Keyhani S, Steigerwald S, Ishida J, et al. Risks and benefits of marijuana use: a national survey of U.S. adults. Ann Intern Med 2018;169(5):282–90.

29. NIDA. Marijuana drugfacts. 2019. Available at: https://www.drugabuse.gov/publications/drugfacts/marijuana. Accessed May 16, 2021.

30. Hackam DG. Cannabis and stroke: systematic appraisal of case reports. Stroke. 2015;46(3):852–6.

31. Grant I, Gonzalez R, Carey CL, et al. Non-acute (residual) neurocognitive effects of cannabis use: a meta-analytic study. J Int Neuropsychol Soc 2003;9(5):679–89.

32. Auer R, Vittinghoff E, Yaffe K, et al. Association between lifetime marijuana use and cognitive function in middle age: the coronary artery risk development in young adults (cardia) study. JAMA Intern Med 2016;176(3):352–61.

33. Choi NG, DiNitto DM, Marti CN. Older-adult marijuana users and ex-users: comparisons of sociodemographic characteristics and mental and substance use disorders. Drug Alcohol Depend. 2016;165:94–102.

34. SAMHSA. Prescription medication misuse and abuse among older adults. Substance Abuse and Mental Health Services Administration; 2012.

35. Odani S, Lin LC, Nelson JR, et al. Misuse of prescription pain relievers, stimulants, tranquilizers, and sedatives among U.S. older adults aged ≥50 years. Am J Prev Med 2020;59(6):860–72.

36. Schepis TS, Simoni-Wastila L, McCabe SE. Prescription opioid and benzodiazepine misuse is associated with suicidal ideation in older adults. Int J Geriatr Psychiatry 2019;34(1):122–9.

37. Lehmann SW, Fingerhood M. Substance-use disorders in later life. N Engl J Med 2018;379(24):2351–60.

38. Huhn AS, Strain EC, Tompkins DA, et al. A hidden aspect of the U.S. opioid crisis: rise in first-time treatment admissions for older adults with opioid use disorder. Drug Alcohol Depend 2018;193:142–7.

39. Rosen D, Engel RJ, Hunsaker AE, et al. Just say know: an examination of substance use disorders among older adults in gerontological and substance abuse journals. Soc Work Public Health 2013;28(3–4):377–87.

40. Han BH. Aging, multimorbidity, and substance use disorders: the growing case for integrating the principles of geriatric care and harm reduction. Int J Drug Policy. 2018;58:135–6.

41. Fink A, Beck JC, Wittrock MC. Informing older adults about non-hazardous, hazardous, and harmful alcohol use. Patient Educ Couns 2001;45(2):133–41.
42. Blow FC, Bartels SJ, Brockmann LM, et al. Evidence-based practices for preventing substance abuse and mental health problems in older adults Older Americans Substance Abuse and Mental Health Technical Assistance Center.
43. Rimer BK, Orleans CT. Tailoring smoking cessation for older adults. Cancer 1994; 74(7 Suppl):2051–4.
44. Henley SJ, Asman K, Momin B, et al. Smoking cessation behaviors among older U.S. Adults Prev Med Rep 2019;16:100978.
45. CDC. About cdc's opioid prescribing guideline. 2021. Available at: https://www.cdc.gov/drugoverdose/prescribing/guideline.html. Accessed May 17, 2021.
46. Schlenk EA, Dunbar-Jacob J, Engberg S. Medication non-adherence among older adults: a review of strategies and interventions for improvement. J Gerontol Nurs 2004;30(7):33–43.
47. Opondo D, Eslami S, Visscher S, et al. Inappropriateness of medication prescriptions to elderly patients in the primary care setting: a systematic review. PLoS One 2012;7(8):e43617.
48. Harley DA, Hancock MT. Substance use disorders intervention with lgbt elders. Handbook of LGBT elders: an interdisciplinary approach to principles, practices, and policies. New York, NY, US: Springer Science + Business Media; 2016. p. 473–90.
49. Afuseh E, Pike CA, Oruche UM. Individualized approach to primary prevention of substance use disorder: age-related risks. Substance Abuse Treat Prev Policy. 2020;15(1):58.
50. SAMHSA. Screening, brief intervention, and referral to treatment (sbirt). 2017. Available at: https://www.samhsa.gov/sbirt. Accessed May 17, 2021.
51. MBHP. Commonly used substance use disorder screening instruments. Massachusetts Behavioral Health Partnership. MassHealth PCC Plan; 2020.
52. SAMHSA. Systems-level implementation of screening, brief intervention, and referral to treatment. Rockville, MD: Substance Abuse and Mental Health Services Administration: Substance Abuse and Mental Health Services Administration; 2013.
53. NIH. Screening tools and prevention. 2019. Available at: https://www.drugabuse.gov/nidamed-medical-health-professionals/screening-tools-prevention. Accessed 3 July, 2021.
54. Piper ME, McCarthy DE, Baker TB. Assessing tobacco dependence: a guide to measure evaluation and selection. Nicotine Tob Res 2006;8(3):339–51.
55. Fiellin DA, Reid MC, O'Connor PG. Screening for alcohol problems in primary care: a systematic review. Arch Intern Med 2000;160(13):1977–89.
56. Purath J, Keck A, Fitzgerald CE. Motivational interviewing for older adults in primary care: a systematic review. Geriatr Nurs 2014;35(3):219–24.
57. Cummings SM, Cooper RL, Cassie KM. Motivational interviewing to affect behavioral change in older adults. Res Soc Work Pract 2008;19(2):195–204.

Moving?

Make sure your subscription moves with you!

To notify us of your new address, find your **Clinics Account Number** (located on your mailing label above your name), and contact customer service at:

Email: **journalscustomerservice-usa@elsevier.com**

800-654-2452 (subscribers in the U.S. & Canada)
314-447-8871 (subscribers outside of the U.S. & Canada)

Fax number: **314-447-8029**

Elsevier Health Sciences Division
Subscription Customer Service
3251 Riverport Lane
Maryland Heights, MO 63043

*To ensure uninterrupted delivery of your subscription, please notify us at least 4 weeks in advance of move.